EAT TO LIVE COOKBOOK

EAT TO LIVE COOKBOOK

200 DELICIOUS NUTRIENT-RICH RECIPES
for Fast and Sustained Weight Loss,
Reversing Disease, and Lifelong Health

Joel Fuhrman, M.D.

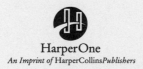

HarperOne
An Imprint of HarperCollinsPublishers

HarperOne

A number of these recipes were originally published in
Eat to Live by Joel Fuhrman, M.D., and are reprinted here by permission of
Little, Brown and Company, a division of Hachette Book Group, Inc.

EAT TO LIVE COOKBOOK: *200 Delicious Nutrient-Rich Recipes for Fast and Sustained
Weight Loss, Reversing Disease, and Lifelong Health.* Copyright © 2013 by Joel Fuhrman, M.D..
All rights reserved. Printed in the United States of America. No part of this book
may be used or reproduced in any manner whatsoever without written permission
except in the case of brief quotations embodied in critical articles and reviews.
For information address HarperCollins Publishers,
10 East 53rd Street, New York, NY 10022.

HarperCollins books may be purchased for educational, business, or sales
promotional use. For information please email the Special Markets Department
at SPsales@harpercollins.com.

HarperCollins website: http://www.harpercollins.com

HarperCollins®, 📖®, and HarperOne™ are trademarks of HarperCollins Publishers

Library of Congress Cataloging-in-Publication Data is available upon request.

ISBN 978–0–06–230995–2

13 14 15 16 17 RRD(H) 10 9 8 7 6 5 4 3 2 1

WELCOME

Congratulations on being part of the Eat to Live family, a rapidly growing army of individuals who embrace a nutritarian lifestyle. This ideal diet-style can both maintain our ideal weight and push the envelope of human longevity. Consuming the healthiest foods on the planet gives the best results: most effective disease reversal, disease protection, longevity enhancement, and the end of dieting.

Eating healthfully also allows us to derive the maximum pleasure and enjoyment out of life. When we eat right, over time, our tastes are modified and we truly enjoy and prefer natural foods. Plus, when we know we are eating for health, we feel emotionally and intellectually secure in our health destiny, which further enhances our appreciation of the food we eat.

I have written this cookbook with the intent of taking the world's healthiest foods and making them even more delicious. These recipes come from my home to yours.

From my family to yours, I wish you the best of health, and a long and pleasurable life.

Joel Fuhrman, M.D.

TABLE OF CONTENTS

INTRODUCTION

EAT TO LIVE IN A NUTSHELL

Eat to Live is a mind-set, a lifestyle, and the title of my *New York Times* #1 bestselling book, *Eat to Live*. When you eat to live, you seek foods, recipes, and menus that are nutrient-rich, so the body is supplied with its nutritional needs for optimum health, disease prevention, and maximum lifespan.

If you want to maintain your good health and enjoy life to the fullest as you age, the secret lies in what you feed your body. Following a plant-based, nutrient-dense diet also enables you to lose weight and keep it off permanently—without hunger or deprivation.

If you want to throw away your medications and recover from chronic illnesses, such as heart disease, high blood pressure, and diabetes (all examples of common illnesses that are more effectively treated with nutritional intervention than drugs or surgery), then the Eat to Live lifestyle is the most effective approach.

Uncovering the cause of a disease, when possible, rather than covering up symptoms with medications, always results in a more favorable outcome. When you maximize nutrients and minimize calories, you become disease-resistant. Countless studies have shown a relationship between nutrition and calories and your longevity and health potential. The majority of Americans ultimately die from their destructive nutritional extravagances.

The most important building block of health is nutrition. Without superior nutrition, your ability to live life to the fullest is limited. Scientific studies reveal that high-nutrient foods such as vegetables, fruits, beans, nuts, and seeds contain vitamins, minerals, and phytochemicals that work in synergy to allow us to achieve the best possible health and immunity from disease. Some of these nutrients are well known while others have yet to be identified. Unfortunately, most of modern society lives on a low-nutrient diet of empty-calorie, processed, refined foods and high-fat, fiberless animal products. It is no wonder we have an overweight, disease-ridden population dying prematurely due to nutritional ignorance.

All of my dietary advice is based on eating larger quantities of nutrient-rich foods and fewer foods with minimal nutritional value. An optimum diet supplies fourteen different vitamins, twenty-five different minerals, and more than one thousand phytochemicals. These plant-based chemicals have profound effects on human cell function and the immune system. The foods that are naturally rich in these nutrients are also high in fiber and water and are naturally low in calories. They provide what your body needs to maximize its self-healing and self-repairing mechanisms.

Nutrient-rich foods are almost always low-calorie foods.
I use a simple formula to express my eating style:

H = N/C

Health = **N**utrients/**C**alories

*Your health is predicted by your nutrient intake
divided by your intake of calories.*

H=N/C is a concept I call my health equation. It stresses the importance of focusing on the nutrient density of your diet. If your nutrient intake is low and your calories are high, your health will be only a fraction of what it could be if you were consuming a high level of nutrients in each calorie.

Food supplies both nutrients and calories (energy). All calories come from only three elements: carbohydrates, fats, and proteins. Nutrients, on the other hand, come from noncaloric food factors, including vitamins, minerals, fiber, and phytochemicals. These noncaloric nutrients are vitally important for your well-being. The key to good health and achieving your ideal body weight is to eat predominantly those foods that have a high proportion of nutrients (noncaloric food factors) to calories (carbohydrates, fats, and proteins).

Our society has evolved to a level of economic sophistication that allows us to eat ourselves to death. A diet centered on milk, cheese, pasta, bread, fried foods, and sugar-filled snacks and drinks lays the groundwork for obesity, cancer, heart disease, diabetes, and autoimmune disease. Although these foods are certainly harmful, that is not the whole problem. The other important issue is what we are *not* eating.

When we evaluate the standard American diet, we find the calories coming from phytochemical-rich foods, such as fresh fruits, vegetables, beans, intact whole grains, raw nuts, and seeds, are less than 13 percent of the total caloric intake. This danger-

As I explain in my book *Super Immunity*:

"Super Immunity" can be best defined as the body's immune system working to its fullest potential. Modern science has advanced to the point where we have evidence that the right raw materials and nutritional factors can double or triple the protective power of the immune system. Superior nutrition is the secret to super immunity. We are dependent on the quality of whole foods grown from the earth to sustain us: the health of the food we eat ultimately determines our own health.

ously low intake of unrefined plant foods guarantees weakened immunity to disease, frequent illnesses, and a shorter lifespan. Until we address this deficiency, we will never win the war on cancer, heart disease, diabetes, and other degenerative diseases.

Many accept that disease is the result of genetics or luck. The reality is that the vast majority of us bear the responsibility for our health through our dietary choices. Nutrition, exercise, and environment simply overwhelm genetics. Poor food choices are the largest cause of disease and premature death.

Vegetables and fruits protect against all types of cancers when consumed in large enough quantities. This is documented by hundreds of scientific studies. The most prevalent cancers in our country are mostly plant-food-deficiency diseases.

Numerous diet plans call for counting calories, eliminating some foods, and adding others, but only this one asks you to strive for more micronutrients in your diet. This diet-style does not require deprivation. There is no calorie counting, portion-size measuring, or weighing involved. You eat as much as you want and, over time, you

• DON AND HIS WIFE •

After fighting a losing battle with diabetes on Glucophage, Actos, and Glyburide, and not wanting to start insulin injections, I wanted to learn about better nutrition, which led me and my wife, who also has diabetes, to Dr. Fuhrman. Together, we learned about his life-changing and life-saving nutritarian plan. I am now off medication. My energy level is better than I can remember, and my A1C is running six. That's down from eleven—all without medication. My wife has lost 34 pounds, and, like me, she's now medication-free. Thank you, Dr. Fuhrman, for giving us back a quality of life!

will be satisfied with fewer calories. As you consume larger and larger portions of nutrient-dense unprocessed foods, your appetite for empty-calorie foods decreases and you gradually lose your addiction to them. At the same time, as the micronutrient quality of your diet increases, your desire to overeat is curtailed.

I have coined the term *nutritarian* to represent a lifestyle that focuses on eating nutrient-rich, natural foods. Those following a nutritarian diet recognize that plant foods have disease-preventive, therapeutic, and life-extending properties. There are many motivations for choosing this lifestyle. You may want to address a current medical concern. You may want to reach and maintain your ideal body weight. You may just want to naturally optimize your health and longevity.

A NUTRITARIAN LIFESTYLE IS ABOUT:

- Eating mainly nutrient-dense, natural plant foods: vegetables, fruits, beans, nuts, and seeds.

- Eating few, if any, animal products (one or two servings per week at most).

- Eating no or almost no foods that are completely empty of nutrients or toxic to the body, such as sugar, sweeteners, white flour, processed foods, and fast foods.

• ROBERT •

I was over 400 pounds. I had high blood pressure, high cholesterol, chronic allergies, osteoarthritis, and rheumatoid arthritis. When my family doctor diagnosed me as a type 2 insulin-resistant diabetic, I finally decided I would no longer be a slave to medicine and poor health. I read all the diabetic literature the doctor gave me and knew right away it was a bunch of nonsense. So I began doing my own research, which eventually led to Dr. Fuhrman. So far I have lost 200 pounds and counting. My cholesterol is normal, my blood pressure is perfect— "low," according to my doctor. My A1C is now under five, and I have no signs of diabetes. I threw away all four of my highly toxic arthritis medicines, and now only need to take the occasional OTC Ibuprofen. My allergies seem to have disappeared, almost entirely. I sold my motorized wheelchair, and now have a full-time job standing on my feet doing manual labor.

Follow these simple nutritarian guidelines:

Include Daily:

1. A large salad

2. At least one ½-cup serving of beans/legumes in soup, salad, or some other dish

3. At least three fresh fruits

4. At least 1 ounce of raw nuts and seeds (if you are trying to lose weight, limit to 1 ounce)

5. At least one large (double-size) serving of cooked green vegetables

Avoid:

1. Red meat and all barbecued, processed, and cured meats

2. Fried foods

3. Full-fat dairy (cheese, ice cream, butter, whole milk, and 2% milk) and trans fat (margarine)

4. Soft drinks, sugar, and artificial sweeteners

5. White rice and white-flour products

This cookbook provides a selection of recipes designed to complement my dietary recommendations. These recipes have been developed to optimize micronutrient density, diversity, and completeness. In addition to the well-known vitamins and minerals, they provide hundreds of other phytonutrients that are important for maximizing immune function, preventing cancer and other diseases, and increasing longevity.

These are some of my favorites and they have become popular with my readers, patients, and participants in my Member Support Center (see DrFuhrman.com /members). If you can eat delicious food that will grant you improved health, ideal weight, disease protection, and a longer life, why choose bad food and poor health? If you think healthy food cannot taste good, then try these recipes. What you may find is that food tastes even more delicious when it makes you the healthiest you can be.

THE BEST INGREDIENTS

VEGETABLES TAKE THE PRIZE

Vegetables, especially green leafy vegetables, win the nutrient density prize. The concentration of vitamins, minerals, phytochemicals, and antioxidants per calorie in vegetables is the highest, by far, of any food. Research shows that vegetable consumption is the most important factor in preventing chronic disease and premature death. Unfortunately, the modern American diet is extremely low in natural vegetation, especially vegetables. It is not slightly deficient in just a handful of micronutrients; it is grossly deficient in hundreds of important plant-derived, immunity-building compounds.

Eating a large amount of greens and other colorful vegetables is the secret weapon to achieve great health. They are low in calories and high in life-extending nutrients. Eat these foods in unlimited quantities and think big. Try to eat a pound of raw vegetables and a pound of cooked vegetables each day. If you can't eat this much don't force yourself, but the idea is to completely rethink what constitutes a portion.

Include lots of salads and raw vegetables in your daily meals. Consuming salads is an effective strategy for weight control. I have treated thousands of patients and have observed that the more salad they eat, the more weight they lose. When you add one of my delicious fruit-, nut-, or avocado-based dressings to your salad, the monounsaturated fats in the dressing increase the body's ability to absorb the anticancer compounds in the raw vegetables. The powerful combination of raw vegetables and healthful dressings makes salad a health food top star.

All vegetables contain protective micronutrients and phytochemicals, but cruciferous vegetables are especially powerful. They are loaded with disease-protecting micronutrients and powerful compounds that promote detoxification and prevent cancer. Cruciferous vegetables have a unique chemical composition: They have sulfur-containing compounds that are responsible for their pungent or bitter flavors. When their cell walls are broken by blending or chopping, a chemical reaction occurs that converts these sulfur-containing compounds into isothiocyanates, an array of compounds with proven and powerful immunity-boosting effects and anticancer activity.

Methods of preparation and cooking affect the absorbability of isothiocyanates (ITCs). Chop, chew, blend, or juice cruciferous vegetables for maximum production of ITCs. They are not pre-formed in the plant; they are made when the plant cell walls are chewed or crushed. The more cell walls that are broken, the more enzymes are released to catalyze the reaction that produces these compounds. Cooking does not destroy the activity and functions of ITCs; it only deactivates the myrosinase enzyme catalyzing their formation. That means if you blend, crush, chop, or juice the greens while they're raw and then put the blended or chopped greens into a stew or soup to cook, you will still have those functioning and beneficial compounds present after cooking.

Onions and mushrooms add great flavor to all kinds of dishes and also have well-documented anticancer and immunity-building properties. Add them to soups, stews, stir-fries, and other vegetable recipes. The allium family of vegetables, which includes onions, garlic, leeks, shallots, chives, and scallions, contains anticancer, anti-inflammatory, and antioxidant compounds. This protection is thought to be due to their organosulfur compounds, which are released when the vegetables are chopped, crushed, or chewed.

CRUCIFEROUS VEGETABLES

Arugula	Cauliflower	Radishes
Bok choy	Collard greens	Red cabbage
Broccoli	Horseradish	Rutabaga leaf
Broccoli rabe	Kale	Swiss chard
Brussels sprouts	Kohlrabi	Turnip greens
Cabbage	Mustard greens	Watercress

Cooked mushrooms contain many unique disease-fighting compounds that are just beginning to be understood. They empower the body to react quickly and powerfully when we are exposed to disease-causing pathogens, such as viruses and bacteria. They also contain compounds called aromatase inhibitors, which help to reduce the risk of breast cancer. As a safety precaution, mushrooms should always be cooked since some animal studies have reported toxic effects of raw mushrooms.

Frozen vegetables are a convenient option. They are rich in micronutrients because they are picked ripe and flash-frozen right on or near the farm. Feel free to substitute frozen vegetables in any of your recipes.

Many metal cans are lined with a BPA-containing resin. BPA (Bisphenol A), is a chemical linked to a number of negative health effects. I recommend that people avoid canned tomato products because tomatoes are acidic and a significant amount of BPA could leach into the food. Use fresh tomatoes or tomatoes packaged in BPA-free cartons. Pomi brand, for example, offers both chopped and strained tomatoes in this type of packaging. Look for tomato paste packaged in glass jars such as the Bionaturæ brand. I recommend purchasing the best fresh tomatoes during the tomato growing season and freezing as many pounds as can fit in your freezer. A box freezer in the garage is a great investment; it enables you to store summer berries, tomatoes, and other produce, self-grown or purchased in bulk.

If you are trying to lose weight, eat as many raw vegetables as desired. Cooked green and nongreen nutrient-rich vegetables (such as eggplant, mushrooms, peppers, onions, tomatoes, carrots, and cauliflower) can also be eaten in unlimited quantities.

To get the maximum immune function benefits of cruciferous vegetables, do the following:

1. Chew all cruciferous greens very, very well, trying to crush every cell.
2. Puree, blend, or chop cruciferous vegetables before adding them to soups, stews, or other cooked dishes.
3. When steaming cruciferous vegetables, such as broccoli or cabbage, try to undercook them slightly so they are not too mushy.
4. Add some raw, chopped, cruciferous vegetables to your salad. The enzymes will increase the production of isothiocyanates.

Starchy vegetables include butternut squash, acorn squash, corn, sweet potatoes, yams, white potatoes, and cooked carrots. They are more calorically dense than the nonstarchy vegetables and may need to be limited to one serving daily for those who want to lose weight. Squash has a better nutritional profile and lower glycemic index compared to potato, so it is a better choice if you are overweight or diabetic. Beans, which I discuss later in this chapter, are even more weight-loss and diabetic friendly.

Overcooking green vegetables causes them to lose valuable nutrients. As the vegetables steam, water-soluble nutrients are lost in the cooking water. Overcooking also deactivates the beneficial myrosinase enzyme in cruciferous vegetables.

Do not cook your vegetables longer than the maximum times given in the ranges below.

Recommended Steaming Times for Green Vegetables:
(once water is boiling)

	Range (minutes)
Artichokes, halved, choke removed	16 – 18
Asparagus	8 – 10
Bok choy	6 – 8
Broccoli, stems separated and quartered	10 – 12
Brussels sprouts	10 – 12
Cabbage, quartered, leaves separated	8 – 10
Kale, collards, Swiss chard	6 – 8
Snow peas	6 – 8
String beans	9 – 11
Zucchini	10 – 12

COLORFUL FRUIT

Try to eat at least three fresh fruits per day. Fruit is an excellent nutrient-dense, low-calorie source of vitamins and phytochemicals. Fruit consumption has been shown to offer strong protection against certain cancers, especially oral, esophageal, lung, prostate, and pancreatic cancers. Researchers have discovered unique substances in fruit that can help prevent aging and deterioration of the brain.

Berries are especially rich in beneficial phytochemical compounds. Their high antioxidant content helps to reduce blood pressure and inflammation, prevent DNA damage that leads to cancer, and protect the brain against oxidative damage that can result in degenerative brain diseases. Berries have the highest nutrient to calorie ratio of all the fruits. All berries, including blueberries, blackberries, raspberries, goji berries, and strawberries, are super foods.

Eat a variety of fruits: apples, apricots, bananas, blueberries, cherries, clementines, grapes, kiwis, mangoes, melons, nectarines, oranges, papayas, peaches, pears, pomegranates, raspberries, strawberries, and tangerines. Try some exotic fruits too, if you have the opportunity. If you need to lose weight, use dried fruits only in small amounts as a sweetener in recipes.

Fruit, consumed at its peak of ripeness, is more delicious than any processed, overrefined dessert or treat. Sadly, in the modern world, most people don't have orchards or gardens full of fresh fruit ready to be picked. Most of the fruit we buy at the grocery store has left the garden far behind, having been picked before its prime to avoid shipping damage and storage loss.

To learn how to choose the best fruit, look for color, smell, texture, and weight. Some fruits tell you that they are ripe by their color. As the acidity of a fruit changes, the green chlorophyll breaks down. Fruits such as bananas and apples have bright colors underneath the green chlorophyll layer; the colors show through as the chlorophyll disappears. Bluish-red berries become a deeper, more intense red as they ripen. For bananas, apples, tomatoes, red berries, and cherries, color change is an excellent indication of ripeness.

Smell is especially important when color is not a good indicator of ripeness—for example, with most melons. Chemical changes take place in ripening fruits that cause them to produce pleasant-smelling compounds. Sniff the blossom end of the fruit (the end opposite the stem) and select fruit that has a full, fruity aroma.

As fruits ripen, the substances that hold the cells together break down and convert to water-soluble pectins, which make the fruit become softer, so a gentle squeeze is a good test for ripeness. If a plum is rock hard, it isn't ripe. The squeeze test is especially useful with fruit that doesn't have a hard or thick rind, so squeeze stone fruit, pears, kiwis, and avocados. This doesn't work as well with melons and pineapples, but even with these hard-coated fruits, a little give is a good sign.

Weight can be a good indicator of ripe fruit. If a fruit feels heavy for its size, it generally means that the fruit is at least fully mature, which is a good start for ripeness. A heavy grapefruit or orange, for example, is usually a good one.

Frozen fruit is a convenient substitute when fresh fruit isn't available. The nutritional value of frozen fruit is comparable to that of fresh fruit. Avoid canned choices; they are not as nutritious. Often they have added sweeteners and have lost some of their water-soluble nutrients.

Since fruit is vital to health and well-being, I use fresh and frozen fruits to make delicious desserts that are nourishing and taste great. I have included many delicious and easy fruit recipes in this cookbook to satisfy your sweet tooth and end your meals on a healthy note.

How to Eat a Mango

Choose a mango that is plump, fragrant, and heavy for its size. Mangoes are ripe when you can indent them slightly with your thumb, but avoid mangoes that are so ripe that they are mushy or have brown marks. Unripe (but not green) mangoes will ripen in a few days when left on your counter. Refrigerate a ripe mango to make it last longer.

In the middle of the mango is a large, flat pit. Holding the mango on its side, make an initial slice slightly off center (so you miss the pit). Take another slice on the other side of the mango. You will now have two "cheeks" plus the pit. Score the two cheeks into cubes. When scoring, cut through until your knife reaches the peel, but do not cut through the peel. Scoop out the mango cubes with a large spoon. Dig deeply along the inside of the peel to get out all the fruit. Now take the piece that contains the pit, peel off the skin and cut off the remaining flesh.

GUIDE TO PICKING
THE BEST RIPE FRUIT

APPLES

A ripe apple will be firm and deeply colored. Depending on the variety, there should also be a slight rosy tone. If you want to find apples with the best flavor, buy them during apple season, which spans from late summer to early winter.

AVOCADOS

In the United States, the two common varieties of avocado are usually referred to as California and Florida avocados. The California avocados (also known as Hass avocados) are the ones with pebbly skins that darken as they ripen. The larger ones with the smooth green rinds are Florida avocados. California, or Hass, avocados tend to be richer and creamier and make better guacamole. Florida avocados are lighter-tasting and contain less fat.

The best way to get a perfectly ripe avocado is to buy a hard, unripe one. Unlike most fruits, avocados start to ripen only after they are picked. As they sit in the produce section of the food market, getting bumped and squeezed by potential customers, the softer, riper fruits may develop bruised spots. These unpalatable bruises are hard to detect from the outside, especially on the Hass variety, which turn black as they ripen. Reduce the chances of blemishes by buying a firm avocado and letting it ripen undisturbed in your kitchen. A ripe avocado yields to gentle pressure but is still somewhat firm. One that feels soft may very well be overripe and brown inside. If your avocado is ripe before you are ready to eat it, put it in the refrigerator where it should keep for a few days.

BANANAS

Ripe bananas are, of course, yellow, but it's okay to buy them while they're still green if you don't plan on eating them for a few days. A yellow banana with a few brown spots is at its height of sweetness. If you are freezing bananas for desserts, wait until the banana is at this fully ripened stage and peel it before putting it into the freezer.

BLACKBERRIES

When choosing blackberries, look for deep, evenly colored berries with a nice sheen. A ripe blackberry is deep black; if the berry is red or purple, it is not ripe. They should be plump and dry and should not have dents or bruises. Check the bottom of the container to make sure there isn't leakage from damaged berries.

BLUEBERRIES

Select fresh blueberries that are completely blue, with no tinge of red. A natural shimmery silver coating on the berries is desirable. Blueberries must be ripe when purchased, as they do not continue to ripen after harvesting. Stained or leaking containers are an indication of fruit past its prime.

CANTALOUPE

Be choosy when picking a cantaloupe because they're often picked while still unripe so they're not damaged during shipping. You can spot an unripe cantaloupe by its green tones. Look for a cream-colored cantaloupe—with no green patches—that has a slightly soft end (the end opposite the stem). Give a sniff and choose one that smells sweet but not overly so, which could mean it's too ripe.

CARAMBOLA (STAR FRUIT)

When ripe, star fruit appear mainly bright yellow with tinges of light green. They may have some dark brown along the five ridges. The flesh should still be quite firm to the touch. You can also buy star fruit when it's green and wait for it to ripen; just leave it on your counter for a few days. When overripe, star fruit turns entirely yellow and starts to have brown spots all over.

CHERIMOYA

Cherimoyas are tropical fruits native to South America. They have a white custard-like flesh, green skin, and black seeds. Choose a cherimoya that is green and firm to the touch and allow it to ripen on the counter or in a paper bag until it is slightly soft. The ripe fruit can be cut in half and scooped out with a spoon. Do not eat the seeds or the skin.

FRESH FIGS

Many Americans are only familiar with dried figs, but fresh figs are a delicious treat. Look for fruit that is slightly soft to the touch with no surface breaks in the skin. Fruit with sap coming out of the end opposite the stem is ripe and has a high sugar content. Figs come in all colors from yellow to brown and red to purple, so you need to know what type of fig it is to use color as a ripeness guide. The most commonly grown figs are a golden yellow when ripe. Because they spoil quite easily, refrigerate and plan on using your fresh figs soon after they ripen.

GRAPES

Ripe grapes are firm and smooth and should still be attached to the stem. Green grapes with a yellowish cast will be sweeter, as will deeply colored red and purple grapes.

JACKFRUIT

Although jackfruit is a common sight throughout Asia, in the West it is still largely unknown. It is huge and prickly on the outside with pods or bulbs inside. The fruit is ripe when it turns from green to yellow. Though it has a notoriously bad smell when ripening, the sweet bulbs are delicious. Jackfruit can also be purchased frozen or dried.

KIWI

A kiwi is ripe when it gives slightly when pressed. Those that are too hard will not be sweet, while those that are too soft or shriveled may be spoiled or fermented.

MANGOES

Finding a ripe mango can be tricky because they can be yellow, red, green, or orange in color. Those that are ready to eat will usually have a yellow hue and should be slightly soft to the touch. Ripe mangoes also have a sweet aroma near the stem end.

PAPAYAS

Papayas with a red-orange skin are ripe and ready to eat. Those with yellow patches are fine, but will take a few days to ripen. Don't eat papayas that are still green or hard, as they are not fully ripe.

PEARS

Most pears in the supermarket are not ripe, so choose those that are firm but not extremely hard and are free from dark soft spots. Brown speckles are okay and may mean better flavor. Once you get the pears home, leave them on the counter to ripen for a few days.

PERSIMMONS

There are two types of persimmons, astringent and nonastringent. The astringent varieties are delicious when soft and fully ripened but are unpleasant-tasting when eaten sooner.

The most common astringent variety is the heart- or acorn-shaped Hachiya, also called Japanese persimmon or Kaki. It should be eaten when very ripe (completely soft). The fruit has a high tannin content, which makes the immature fruit astringent and unpalatable. The tannin gradually disappears as the fruit matures. When ready to eat, the flesh becomes sweet, aromatic, and almost liquid. A ripe (soft-ripe) persimmon is like a thin skin full of thick jelly. The fruit ripens and softens from the top down, so the trick to enjoying a persimmon is to let it ripen until the wide bottom edge around the leaf is soft. The ripe fruit can then be refrigerated until eaten.

Nonastringent persimmons are shorter, tomato-shaped, and most commonly sold as the Fuyu variety. The Sharon fruit is a type of Fuyu persimmon. These nonastringent persimmons can be consumed when firm and also remain edible when soft.

PINEAPPLES

You can find a ripe pineapple by choosing one that's heavy for its size and has a sweet smell, particularly near the stem. The bottom end should be starting to turn yellow; if it is green throughout, it is typically unripe.

PLUMS

The best plums are those that yield slightly to pressure and have a deep color and a semi-soft tip. Plums that feel firm will ripen in a few days, but avoid those that are rock hard, as they may have been harvested too soon to ever fully ripen.

POMEGRANATES

The ripest pomegranates are found in fall and early winter. When you pick them up, they should feel heavy, an indication they are full of juice and ripe. The skin should be dark or bright red and tight and smooth with no cracks or bruises.

To open and deseed a pomegranate, make a ½-inch cut around its center and then twist back and forth until it splits in two. Hold the half of the pomegranate loosely in your palm and opened fingers with the flat, cut side down. With the other hand, hit all around the top, rounded skin, rotating, smacking, and softening each segment, which pops all the seeds out between your fingers. Once softened, turn the skin inside out to look for remaining kernels to remove, if any.

STRAWBERRIES

Strawberries are ripe when they're a deep red color with a shiny skin. Avoid buying any with green or yellow patches, as they're unripe and won't ripen any further. Most often, it is best to stay away from very large strawberries. Though they look good, their flavor is often inferior to smaller berries.

WATERMELONS

With cut pieces, look for watermelon flesh that is bright red in color. It should be firm and not mushy or watery. Stay clear of watermelon that has white streaks in the flesh, has a pinkish flesh, or is too deeply colored and spoiled. For whole melons, choose a firm, heavy watermelon with a smooth skin, and be sure it has a well-defined yellow area on one side. This is the spot where the watermelon rested while ripening. If it's not there, it means it may have been harvested too soon.

DON'T FORGET THE BEANS

If you have read any of my other books, you know I rank beans among the world's most perfect foods. Beans and greens are the most favorable foods for weight loss, closely linked in the scientific literature with protection against cancer, diabetes, heart disease, stroke, and dementia. They also stabilize blood sugar, blunt your desire for sweets, and help you feel full.

Beans contain both insoluble fiber and soluble fiber and are very high in resistant starch. Although resistant starch is technically a starch, it acts more like fiber and

How to Cook Beans

Beans will generally triple in volume when cooked. One cup of dry beans will yield 3 cups of cooked beans. Sort dried beans before using to pick out any shriveled or broken beans, stones, or debris. Rinse the sorted beans well in cold, running water.

Most dried beans should be soaked before cooking. There are two soaking methods:

- **Regular soak:** Put beans into a large bowl and cover with 2 to 3 inches of water. Set aside at room temperature for 8 hours or overnight. Drain well.

- **Quick soak:** Put beans into a large pot and cover with 2 to 3 inches of water. Bring to a boil and boil briskly for 2 to 3 minutes. Cover, remove from heat, and let sit for 1 hour. Drain well.

After soaking and draining, put beans in a large pot, add water (use a 3:1 ratio; for example, 3 cups of water for 1 cup of beans), and bring beans to a boil. Lower the heat, cover, and simmer, stirring occasionally, until beans are tender when mashed or pierced with a fork. Most beans require about 90 minutes to 2 hours of cooking. Lentils and split peas require 1 hour and should not be soaked prior to cooking. Make sure beans are thoroughly cooked as they are more difficult to digest when undercooked.

Beans may also be cooked in a pressure cooker to reduce cooking time. Put the beans in the pressure cooker with three times as much water as beans. Cook at 15 pounds pressure for 30 minutes for small beans and about 40 minutes for large beans.

"resists digestion." Since it passes through the small intestine undigested, a significant amount of the carbohydrate calories in beans are not absorbed.

Try to eat a cup of cooked beans each day. Consider them your preferred high-carbohydrate food. Among your choices are chickpeas, black-eyed peas, black beans, split peas, lima beans, pinto beans, lentils, red kidney beans, soybeans, cannellini beans, and white beans. Many of my soup and stew recipes contain beans. You can also add them to a salad to make a filling meal. For most of my bean-containing recipes, you can substitute one type of bean for another. No need to do an extra run to the market if you don't have the particular bean called for in the recipe.

If you choose to use canned beans instead of cooking your own dried beans, make sure you select products that are labeled as "low-sodium" or "no-salt-added." Since beans are not an acidic food, there is less concern with BPA (Bisphenol A) from the can lining leaching into the food. You can also choose Eden brand canned beans; they report that they use non-BPA cans. Soft, "cooked" beans are also available in BPA-free box packaging.

SOURCES OF GOOD FAT: NUTS, SEEDS, AND AVOCADOS

High-fat plant foods are rich in the essential fatty acids that your body needs. Nuts, seeds, and avocados are some of nature's ideal foods and are the best source of healthful fats. They increase the absorption of nutrients in vegetables in addition to supplying their own spectrum of micronutrients, including plant sterols, which help to reduce cholesterol.

The villain is not fat in general, but rather oils, saturated fats, trans fats, and the fats consumed in processed foods. Fats from nuts, seeds, and avocados are rich in antioxidants and phytochemicals and offer unique health benefits. Nuts and seeds are strongly protective against heart disease and provide omega-3 fats. They are also a plant-food source of protein.

Remember the four high-omega-3 seeds and nuts:

Flax • Chia • Hemp • Walnuts

A Word About Food Allergies

You can still follow a high-nutrient diet-style even if you have food allergies. Remember, the basic concept is to select the foods that have the highest nutrient-per-calorie ratio. This can be done even if you need to avoid certain foods.

If you are allergic to nuts, you can substitute raw seeds: sunflower seeds, unhulled sesame seeds, ground flax seeds, and chia seeds.

In soup and salad dressing recipes that involve blending cashews or almonds, you can generally substitute raw sunflower seeds or sunflower seed butter. Unhulled sesame seeds or raw tahini are other options, but because they are stronger in flavor, you should start off with a lower amount than the original recipe calls for and adjust according to your taste.

Researchers have found that including nuts and seeds in your diet can help you lose weight. Although nuts and seeds are not low in calories and are relatively high in fat, their consumption may actually satisfy hunger and suppress appetite. I find that eating a small amount of nuts or seeds helps dieters feel satiated, stay with the program and have more success at long-term weight loss. If you are significantly overweight, eat only an ounce (about ¼ cup) of nuts or seeds a day; if you are thin, physically active, pregnant, or nursing, you may eat 2 to 4 ounces, according to your caloric needs.

Seeds give you all the advantages of nuts, plus more. They are generally higher in protein than nuts and have many additional important nutrients, making them a particularly wonderful food.

Flax, chia, and hemp seeds provide omega-3 fatty acids, which are essential for good health. Flax, sesame, and chia seeds are also rich in anticancer lignans. These

• LACEY •

I dealt with debilitating migraines for more than 13 years, getting about three to four per week. My symptoms included vomiting, blurred vision, sensitivity to sunlight, and extreme pain. After years of prescription pain killers, dozens of doctors, every test imaginable, and absolutely no success, I read *Eat to Live* and made a drastic decision to completely change my dietary habits. Since the day I started—February 1, 2011—I have been 100 percent migraine free and have lost 40 pounds.

plant compounds bind to estrogen receptors and interfere with the cancer-promoting effects of estrogen on breast tissue. They also have strong antioxidant effects.

Pumpkin seeds also contain omega-3 fats, as well as vitamin E, iron, and other minerals. Sunflower seeds are high in protein and minerals. Sesame seeds are very high in calcium and supply a highly absorbable form of vitamin E.

Flax seeds should be ground before using, as they are just too difficult to chew. Ground flax seeds oxidize and become rancid faster so I recommend that you buy flax seeds whole and then grind them at home. Store your flax seeds in the freezer to prevent them from spoiling.

Eat nuts and seeds raw or only lightly toasted or roasted, because the roasting process alters their beneficial nutrients. Commercially packaged nuts and seeds are also frequently cooked in oil and heavily salted. If you tire of eating nuts and seeds raw, try lightly toasting them at home. This does not deplete their beneficial properties and will add some variety. Bake in a 250°F oven for about 20 minutes, stirring occasionally, until they are very lightly browned. Do not heavily brown them, as this causes carcinogenic compounds called acrylamides to be produced.

Consume nuts and seeds with your meals, not as snacks, because they facilitate the absorption of essential phytochemicals from other foods. Many of the recipes in this cookbook use these disease-fighting foods to make delicious salad dressings, dips, and creamy soups. Choose from the wide variety of nuts and seeds: almonds, cashews,

I have created an acronym to help you remember the
super foods that you should include in your diet every day.
G-BOMBS—Greens, Beans, Onions, Mushrooms, Berries, and Seeds—
are the most powerful longevity-promoting, immunity-strengthening foods.
More details about these amazing foods can be found in my
New York Times bestselling book, *Super Immunity*.

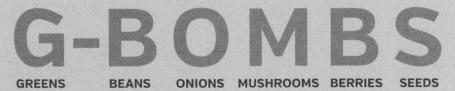

G-BOMBS

GREENS   BEANS   ONIONS   MUSHROOMS   BERRIES   SEEDS

walnuts, pecans, hazelnuts, macadamias, pignoli, pistachios, sesame seeds, sunflower seeds, pumpkin seeds, hemp seeds, chia seeds, and flax seeds. Pay extra attention to include some walnuts, flax, hemp, and chia seeds in your diet because they contain the highest amounts of omega-3 fats.

WHOLE GRAINS ARE NOT SUPER FOODS

Grain products are the least nutrient-dense foods of the seed family and do not show the powerful protection against disease that is apparent in the scientific studies on vegetables, beans, onions, mushrooms, berries, and seeds. Therefore, they should be consumed in smaller caloric amounts. Grains do not contain enough nutrients per calorie to form the major part of your diet.

Make sure the grains you do include in your diet are 100% whole grain. Whole-grain products contain all the essential parts and naturally occurring nutrients of the entire grain seed. All of the original kernel—the bran, germ, and endosperm—are present in a whole grain. Whole grains include barley, buckwheat (kasha), millet, old-fashioned oats, quinoa, spelt, and brown, black, and wild rice. The intact (unground) whole grains and the more coarsely ground grains that are absorbed into the bloodstream more slowly, are healthier, and curtail appetite more effectively.

Bread products made with sprouted grains are good choices. Wheat kernels, as well as other grains, such as millet, barley, and oats, are allowed to sprout and are then ground up and baked into bread. Sprouted grains are a favorable source of grain as

• JEFF •

The past two months have been incredible! At the start of Dr. Fuhrman's program, I weighed 335 pounds with blood pressure around 160/110. I was taking several blood pressure medications. I was barely fitting into my 52-inch-waist pants. On Nov. 2, my cardiologist told me I had developed atrial fibrillation, probably due to severe obstructive sleep apnea. That's when I read *Eat to Live* and started on the program. Two months later, I have lost 40 pounds and 4 inches off my waist. My blood pressure is under control and my a-fib is gone. I still have a long way to go, but I now know how to get there. It is not exaggerating to say that Dr. Fuhrman saved my life!

they are coarsely ground and have an improved nutrient and glycemic profile. Many stores carry sprouted-grain breads such as Ezekiel and Manna brands in their freezer sections.

When choosing a whole-grain bread, pita, or wrap, read the ingredient list to make sure it is 100% whole grain. It should list "whole" grain as the first ingredient. If more than one grain is used, they should all be whole grains. Just because a bread product claims to be multigrain (twelve grain, nine grain, etc.) or whole wheat, it does not mean it is 100% whole grain. It may be made of various grains that are all refined or may just include a small amount of whole-wheat flour, so make sure to read the ingredient list thoroughly.

LIMIT ANIMAL PRODUCTS

All animal products, including meat, fish, and dairy, are low (or completely lacking) in the nutrients that protect us against cancer and heart attacks. Plant foods–not animal foods–contain fiber, antioxidants, and hundreds of phytochemicals. Animal products are rich in substances that scientific investigations have shown to be associated with the incidence of cancer and heart disease: saturated fat, cholesterol, and arachidonic acid. Convincing science has also demonstrated that diets higher in animal protein promote cancer. Animal protein, because it has a high biological value, and because the protein is highly concentrated, promotes the rise of cancer-promoting hormones within the body, especially IGF-1 (insulin-like growth factor-1).

Almost all Americans get enough protein daily. In fact, the average American consumes over 100 grams of protein each day, about 50 percent more than the recommended daily amount. It is true that a certain lifestyle, one involving vigorous and regular physical workouts, requires additional protein, but the increased need for protein is proportional to the increased need for extra calories burned from exercise. As exercise increases our appetite, we increase our caloric intake accord-

It is best never to eat until you are full. Stop eating before you feel uncomfortable. Stand up and walk around three-quarters of the way through a meal to make sure you are not overeating.

ingly, and our protein intake increases proportionally. If we meet the increased caloric demand from heavy exercise with a variety of natural plant foods, vegetables, beans, whole grains, nuts, and seeds, we will get the precise amount of extra protein needed.

You do not need to rely on animal products for protein. A typical assortment of vegetables, beans, whole grains, nuts, and seeds supplies about 35 grams of protein per 1,000 calories.

I recommend limiting animal products, including cheese, yogurt, and milk, to 10 percent or less of your daily caloric intake. Ideally, if you do include animal products in your diet, limit the serving size to 2 ounces and not more than three times a week. Do not make animal products the focus of the meal. Think of them as a garnish, condiment, or flavoring agent. Two ounces of chopped or shredded seafood or fowl is enough to impart flavor without driving up cancer-promoting hormones.

When consuming animal products, choose fat-free dairy, eggs, clean wild fish, and organic meat and poultry. Avoid processed and barbecued meats, luncheon meats, bacon, hot dogs, and any pickled, darkened, or blackened animal products.

MISCONCEPTIONS ABOUT OLIVE OIL

No oil should be considered a health food. All oil, including olive oil, is 100 percent fat and contains 120 calories per tablespoon. Oil is high in calories, low in nutrients, and contains no fiber. Add a few tablespoons of oil to your salad or vegetable dish and you've added hundreds of wasted calories. It is the perfect food to help you put on unwanted and unhealthful pounds.

Oil is a processed food. When oil is chemically extracted from a whole food (such as olives, nuts, or seeds), it leaves behind (loses) the vast majority of micronutrients and becomes a fragmented food that contains little more than empty calories.

Foods rich in monounsaturated fats, like olive oil, are less harmful than foods full of saturated fats and trans fats, but being less harmful does not make them "healthful." The beneficial effects of the Mediterranean diet are not due to the consumption of olive oil; they are due to antioxidant-rich foods, including vegetables, fruits, and beans, as well as lots of onions and garlic. Eating a lot of any kind of oil means you're eating a lot of empty calories, which leads to excess weight and can also lead to diabetes, high blood pressure, stroke, heart disease, and many forms of cancer.

You can add a little bit of olive oil to your diet if you are thin and exercise a lot. However, the more oil you add, the more you are lowering the nutrient-per-calorie density of your diet, and that is not your objective, as it will not promote health and longevity.

THE ANDI FOOD SCORING SYSTEM

To illustrate which foods have the highest nutrient-per-calorie density, I have ranked the nutrient density of many common foods in my Aggregate Nutrient Density Index, or ANDI. These scores rank a variety of foods based on how many nutrients they deliver to your body for each calorie consumed. The highest score is 1,000. Food labels list only a few nutrients, but my scores are based on twenty-eight important micronutrients plus other properties. The scores are a simple way to help identify and eat larger amounts of nutrient-rich foods. The higher the scores and the greater percentage of those foods in your diet, the better your health will be. ANDI is an easy visualization of which foods are the most beneficial to eat and how foods compare to one another in nutrient density. The table on page 28 contains a sample of my ANDI scores.

It is important to achieve micronutrient diversity, not just a high level of a few isolated micronutrients. Micronutrient adequacy means obtaining enough of all the beneficial nutrients, not merely higher amounts of a select few while other micronutrient needs go unfulfilled.

Eating a variety of plant foods is the key to achieving micronutrient diversity. Consider onions and cooked mushrooms to illustrate this concept. They may not contain the highest amounts of vitamins and minerals, but they contain a significant amount of unique protective phytochemicals that are not found in other foods, such as cancer-protective aromatase inhibitors, organosulfides, and angiogenesis inhibitors. A small amount of mushrooms and onions in the diet adds more micronutrient diversity, even though they are not the highest-scoring foods when we add up all their micronutrients.

Focus not only on the nutritional quality of what you eat, but also on the proper spectrum of foods that supply the full symphonic orchestra of human requirements. This means that certain plant foods, such as onions, seeds, mushrooms, berries, beans, and tomatoes, aid in achieving micronutrient quality and contribute to the numerator in my H=N/C equation, even though they might not have the most nutrients per calorie.

You achieve superior health and permanent weight control by eating more nutrient-rich foods and fewer high-calorie, low-nutrient foods. This works because the more high-nutrient foods you consume, the fewer low-nutrient foods you desire.

How do the foods you eat rate?

DR. FUHRMAN'S **ANDI** SCORES

Kale 1,000	Pomegranates. 119	Walnuts. 30
Collard greens 1,000	Cantaloupe. 118	Bananas 30
Mustard greens. . . .1,000	Onions. 109	Whole-wheat bread . . 30
Watercress 1,000	Flax seeds 103	Almonds 28
Swiss chard 895	Orange 98	Avocado 28
Bok choy. 865	Edamame 98	Brown rice 28
Spinach. 707	Cucumber. 87	White potato 28
Arugula 604	Tofu 82	Low-fat plain yogurt . . 28
Romaine 510	Sesame seeds 74	Cashews 27
Brussels sprouts 490	Lentils 72	Oatmeal 26
Carrots 458	Peaches 65	Chicken breast. 24
Cabbage 434	Sunflower seeds 64	Ground beef, 85% lean . . . 21
Broccoli. 340	Kidney beans 64	Feta cheese 20
Cauliflower. 315	Green peas. 64	White bread 17
Bell peppers. 265	Cherries 55	Estimated ANDI without fortification 9
Mushrooms 238	Pineapple 54	White pasta 16
Asparagus 205	Apple 53	Estimated ANDI without fortification 11
Tomato 186	Mango. 53	French fries 12
Strawberries 182	Peanut butter 51	Cheddar cheese 11
Sweet potato 181	Corn. 45	Apple juice 11
Zucchini 164	Pistachio nuts 37	Olive oil 10
Artichoke 145	Shrimp. 36	Vanilla ice cream. 9
Blueberries. 132	Salmon 34	Corn chips 7
Iceberg lettuce 127	Eggs. 34	Cola 1
Grapes. 119	Milk, 1%. 31	

TO MAKE IT EASIER FOR YOU TO FIND THE VERY BEST FOODS, I'VE LISTED MY TOP 25 SUPER FOODS

1. Collard, mustard, turnip greens 1,000
2. Kale 1,000
3. Watercress 1,000
4. Swiss chard 895
5. Bok choy 865
6. Cabbage (all varieties) 434–715
7. Spinach 707
8. Arugula 604
9. Lettuce (Boston, romaine, red & green leaf) 367–585
10. Brussels sprouts 490
11. Carrots 458
12. Broccoli 340
13. Cauliflower 315
14. Bell peppers, red and green 240–270
15. Mushrooms 238
16. Tomatoes 186
17. Berries (all varieties) 132–182
18. Asparagus 205
19. Pomegranates 119
20. Grapes 119
21. Cantaloupe 118
22. Onions 109
23. Beans (all varieties) 43–98
24. Seeds (flax, hemp, chia, sesame, pumpkin, sunflower) 39–103
25. Nuts (all varieties) 26–60

There is more to being a super food than having a high ANDI score. We still require nutritional diversity and some highly recommended foods may not be high in USDA-measured nutrients, but have other overwhelming qualities that do not give them a high ANDI. Take onions and mushrooms, for example: they contain powerful anticancer phytochemicals, but are not high enough in vitamins and minerals to earn a very high ANDI. Also, the health-giving properties of nuts and seeds, with their beneficial fats, sterols, and stanols, are not registered adequately in the ANDI because their calorie count is high. We can't just eat high-ANDI, low-calorie vegetables anyway or we would be hungry all the time and get too thin. So ANDI is a valuable tool, but not the only information one needs.

WHAT'S ON YOUR PLATE?

Today, most health authorities agree that we should add more servings of fruits and vegetables to our diet. I disagree with this approach. It doesn't adequately address the problem. Instead of just adding protective fruits, vegetables, beans, nuts, and seeds to our disease-causing diet, we must make these foods the main focus of the diet itself.

The Choose My Plate icon published by the USDA puts more emphasis on the consumption of vegetables and fruits than the previous Food Guide Pyramid but still falls short of giving the advice people need to optimize their health.

USDA CHOOSE MY PLATE

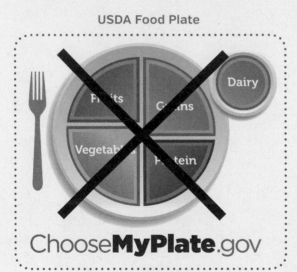

USDA Food Plate

ChooseMyPlate.gov

WARNING: DO NOT CHOOSE THIS PLATE

In the USDA Choose My Plate graphic, foods are grouped in a way that does not make sense. Meat, beans, nuts, and seeds are in the same food group because they are considered protein-rich; however, while nuts, seeds, and beans have been shown to reduce cholesterol levels and heart disease risk, meat is linked to increased risk. Choose My Plate would also lead you to believe that dairy should be consumed on a daily basis. Including milk as its own very prominent group implies that it is an essential part of a healthy diet, which is anything but the truth, especially with the strong association of dairy with negative health consequences, including several cancers. The bottom line is that this plate offers little help for those really wanting to reduce their health risks.

THE NUTRITARIAN FOOD PLATE

I have developed my own Nutritarian Food Plate to illustrate what your plate should really look like. It is comprised of nutrient-rich plant foods according to their nutrient composition and disease-protective properties. Raw and cooked vegetables, fruits, beans, nuts, seeds, and whole grains should fill up almost all of your plate.

Poultry, eggs, dairy, fish, oil, and white potatoes should comprise 10 percent or less of your plate. Cheese, sweets, red meat, processed foods, and white rice and flour should be eaten rarely, if at all. They provide few antioxidants and phytochemicals and decrease the nutrient density of your diet. Significant quantities of "high-protein" foods also drive up hormones linked to higher rates of breast, prostate, and colon cancers.

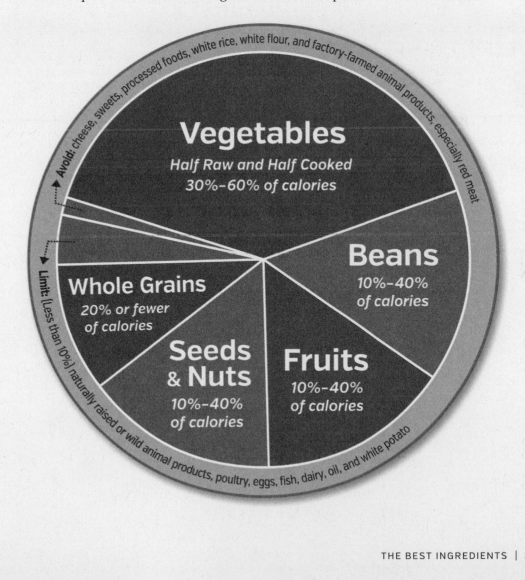

• JILL •

Eight and a half years ago I had a miscarriage that knocked me off my feet. I turned to food for comfort and became an obsessive emotional eater. My weight piled on year after year. While my husband and I continued to try to get pregnant, I was diagnosed with polycystic ovarian syndrome and placed on several medications to regulate my hormones. I spent eight years in and out of an infertility clinic, where doctors ran endless tests and increased my medications. This summer I came to the end of my rope. I knew it was time to make major changes in my lifestyle. I started reading *Eat to Live* one afternoon. Later that evening, I was already making changes in my food choices, which continued the more I read and the more I educated myself on food, nutrition, and health.

I have already lost 85 pounds and am thrilled to report that I am pregnant with a healthy baby. I am continuing to Eat to Live and have no desire to change. I can't wait to teach my child how to do the same.

Thank you, Dr. Fuhrman, thank you times a million!

COOK TO LIVE

Cooking to Live can be simple or gourmet. You do not have to be a chef and have a lot of time to cook wonderful meals. On the other hand, if you do enjoy preparing food, there is no need to stifle your culinary creativity.

I have included a variety of recipes in this cookbook; some are quick and easy and others, developed by world-class chefs, are worthy of the finest gourmet restaurant. Some of the recipes were contributed by participants in the Member Support Center at my website (DrFuhrman.com).

HELPFUL TOOLS AND TECHNIQUES

There are a few tools and techniques that you will find helpful in preparing my *Eat to Live Cookbook* recipes. Take a few minutes to make sure you are familiar with these important basics:

• GOOD KNIFE SET

Invest in a good set of knives and keep them well-sharpened. Sharp knives are safer and easier to use than dull ones. A food chopper is also a time-saver for chopping and dicing vegetables and fruits.

• WOK WITH COVER OR LARGE PAN WITH COVER

Water-sautéing (also called sweating or steam-frying) is used instead of cooking with oil. Water-sautéing is simple and easy to use for stir-fries, sauces, and many other dishes. To water-sauté, heat a skillet, wok, or pan on high heat until water sputters when dropped on the pan. Add a tablespoon or two of water and, when hot, add the vegetables and cook, covering occasionally and adding more water as necessary until tender. Do not add too much water, or the food will be boiled not sautéed. To develop flavor in the onions, garlic, or other vegetables you are cooking, let the pan get dry enough for the food to start to brown just a little before you add additional water. No-salt-added vegetable broth, coconut water, tomatoes, wine, or unsweetened fruit juice may also be used for sautéing stir-fries and vegetable dishes.

● HIGH-POWERED BLENDER

Some of the recipes in this cookbook require a powerful blender. Even though it's an expensive piece of equipment, it is well worth the investment because it produces smooth and creamy salad dressings, sauces, dips, smoothies, sorbets, and blended salads. It is ideal for pureeing vegetables and nuts into soup and grinding nuts and seeds. The Vitamix brand blender is a good choice.

● VEGETABLE JUICER

Although not as critical as a high-powered blender, a vegetable juicer is a useful addition to your kitchen. Fresh-squeezed juice is more flavorful than canned or bottled juice. Using freshly juiced, organic carrots in my soup recipes that call for carrot juice will optimize the flavor of these recipes. Consuming a beverage made from a combination of fresh-squeezed vegetables is an effective way to boost your nutrient consumption.

A juicer is different from a blender. When fruits or vegetables are put into a blender, the end product contains everything that went into the blender, but a juicer will separate the juice from the pulp. With juicing, you retain many of the phytochemicals and other nutrients, but lose some beneficial components like fiber. Juicing should not replace eating fruits and vegetables in your diet, but it is an effective way to increase your nutrient absorption because it allows you to easily consume a lot of nutrients from vegetables.

● PRESSURE COOKER

Steaming vegetables with a pressure cooker preserves more nutrients than regular steaming because the vegetables can be softened in a significantly shorter cooking time, with less water and without excessive heat.

When pressure cooking vegetables, add carrots, garlic, peppers, mushrooms, or onions for more flavor. Do not discard the liquid at the bottom of the pot. It contains valuable water-soluble nutrients. Simply stir it back in with the rest of the veggies before serving. Cooking soups and stews with a pressure cooker produces a healthful and tasty meal in half the time.

SPICES, HERBS, AND CONDIMENTS

Season your foods with fresh or dried herbs and spices instead of salt. They contribute unique flavors as well as color and variety. Experiment with a wide variety of seasoning options and soon you will not even miss the salt you used to pile on your food.

I do not use salt in any of my recipes and I specify low-sodium versions of ingredients, such as store-bought vegetable broth and tomato sauce. Any excess salt added to food, outside of what is contained in natural foods, has the potential to increase your risk of developing disease. High sodium intake is linked to high blood pressure and is predictive of increased incidence of death from heart attacks, strokes, and stomach cancer. A high sodium intake also causes increased loss of calcium in urine, which may influence bone loss and contribute to osteoporosis.

Using a lot of salt in your diet dulls your taste buds and makes you feel that food tastes bland unless it is heavily salted or spiced. It takes some time for one's salt-saturated taste buds to get used to a low-sodium diet. When you avoid processed foods or highly salted foods, your ability to detect and enjoy subtle natural flavors will improve.

I recommend that you keep your overall daily sodium intake under 1,200 mg and preferably under 1,000 mg. Natural foods contain less than 0.5 mg of sodium per calorie. If a serving of food provides 100 calories and contains 400 mg of sodium, it has excessive levels of added salt. Since you get 400–700 mg of sodium daily from natural whole foods, you don't want processed foods to push you over the limit.

When using condiments, mustard and salsa are okay, but choose low-sodium versions that are available in health food stores and many supermarkets. Avoid pickled

Many of the recipes in this book use my VegiZest and MatoZest seasoning blends. These unique vegetable supplements add flavor and provide additional antioxidants and phytochemicals. They contain powerful anticancer foods such as kale, broccoli, spinach, tomato, green tea, and onion.

You can also experiment with other no-salt seasoning blends. There are a variety of products available in the spice section of your market that will provide interesting flavors without adding salt.

foods and olives; they are usually too high in salt. Soy sauce, even low-sodium soy sauce, is high in sodium. I use a small amount of Bragg Liquid Aminos in a few of my recipes, but this product also contains sodium and should only be used in limited quantities.

When cooking without salt, you can increase flavor by adding a moderate level of heat with ingredients such as black pepper, cayenne pepper, or crushed red pepper flakes. Vinegar, or citrus ingredients, such as lemon, lime, or orange, also enhance a recipe. These acidic ingredients activate the same taste receptors as salt. I also like to use raw or roasted garlic to kick up the flavor in my recipes.

Each spice or herb has a distinctive flavor. Consider the flavor of the main ingredient in your recipe. In general, the weaker the flavor of the food, the less seasoning you need to give balance to the recipe. Dried herbs are stronger than fresh herbs because the chemicals that produce the characteristic flavor are more concentrated. Powdered spices are stronger than crumbled spices since they can more easily mix with the food. A useful guide is:

¼ teaspoon powdered = ¾ to 1 teaspoon crumbled = 2 to 3 teaspoons fresh

In dishes with shorter cooking times, crush dried herbs first to release some of the oils. When using fresh herbs, chop the leaves very finely. The more cut surface exposed, the more flavor will be released. Cook heartier herbs—such as thyme, oregano, and sage—along with the other ingredients in the recipe. Add the more tender herbs like basil, parsley, and chives at the end for fresher flavor.

Strong or dominant flavor:
bay leaf, cardamom, curry (a blend of spices), cumin, ginger, pepper, mustard, rosemary, sage

Medium flavor:
basil, cilantro, celery seeds, cumin, dill, fennel, tarragon, garlic, marjoram, mint, oregano, savory, thyme, turmeric

Delicate flavor:
chives, parsley, chervil

Sweet flavor:
cinnamon, cloves, allspice, ginger, cardamom, anise, fennel, mint

Savory flavor:
oregano, tarragon, chives, dill

Peppery flavor:
cayenne pepper, mustard, black pepper, paprika, chili powder
Use with care since their flavors stand out.

Quick Tip:
Avoid packaged foods that contain more milligrams (mg) of sodium than the number of calories.

Spices and herbs can be grouped together based on the strength of their flavor. When using more than one spice or herb, it is usually best not to mix very strong-flavored herbs together. Combine one strong-flavored with one or more milder-flavored herbs to complement both the stronger herb and the food. Medium-flavored seasonings can be used in moderate amounts. Delicate-flavored seasonings may be used in large quantities and can be combined with most other herbs and spices.

FOOD SHOPPING

It is easy to shop for nutrient-dense foods. They are found mostly in the produce aisle. Since it is necessary to consume a variety of fresh fruits and vegetables, I recommend that you shop twice a week. You can use the main shopping trip of the week to stock up on staples and enough produce for three or four days. Your second trip of the week can be a short run to restock fresh fruits and vegetables. You will spend most of your time in the produce, health food, and perhaps frozen food sections. The supermarket is filled with temptation, so try to avoid certain aisles. The center aisles of most stores contain the most heavily processed foods; they should be avoided.

With the exception of unprocessed frozen fruits and vegetables, most foods that come in boxes, bags, and jars are highly processed and low in nutrients per calorie. Don't be misled by the writing on the package. It is essentially advertising and tells you little, if anything, about the nutritional content of the product. The ingredient list contains the most important information. Read it before putting an item into your shopping cart. You will probably end up putting it back on the shelf.

Ingredients are listed on the label according to quantity, in descending order (from most to least) based on weight. This means the first three ingredients in the list are what you are primarily eating. Avoid products with ingredient lists that contain long chemical words that you don't understand. Stay with ingredients you recognize. Avoid foods that list any type of sweetener, such as sugar, sucrose, dextrose, or corn syrup, or use white flour (often called wheat flour) instead of 100% whole-wheat or whole-grain flour. Partially hydrogenated oils are the primary source of trans fats, which have been shown to be potentially more harmful to arteries than saturated fat. If a food lists partially hydrogenated vegetable oil, hydrogenated vegetable oil, or shortening among the ingredients, it contains trans fats.

When looking at labels, be aware of sodium levels. Large amounts of sodium are "hidden" in processed foods, such as pasta sauce and canned soup. If you do buy processed foods, look for products that are labeled "low sodium" or "no salt added." Foods that are labeled as reduced or less sodium are not low sodium. It only means that they contain 25 percent less sodium than the regular product.

SHOULD I BUY ORGANIC PRODUCE?

It is better to eat fruits and vegetables grown and harvested using pesticides than not to eat them at all, but it is also wise to minimize your pesticide exposure.

Every study to date on the consumption of food and its relation to cancer has shown that the more fruits and vegetables people eat, the less cancer and heart disease they have. All these studies were done on people eating conventionally grown, not organic produce. Although the health benefits of eating phytochemical-rich produce greatly outweigh the risks that pesticide residues might pose, recent studies have documented a link between certain diseases and pesticides ingested from foods.

When possible, peel fruits and do not eat potato skins, unless they are organic. If not organically grown, remove and discard the outermost leaves of lettuce and cabbage, as well as other surfaces that cannot be peeled or washed with soap and water or a commercial vegetable wash.

The quality of the food is what makes the dish.

You can have the most incredible combination of seasonings and superb preparation, but if the quality of the ingredients is poor, the dish will miss the mark. The most simple foods are delicious as long as the ingredients are top quality. Don't skimp on quality or freshness.

If you are concerned about pesticides and chemicals, keep in mind that commercially raised animal products, such as dairy, fish, and beef, contain the most toxic pesticide and chemical residues. Because cows and steers eat large amounts of tainted feed, certain pesticides and dangerous chemicals are found in higher concentrations in animal foods. For example, dioxin, which is predominantly found in fatty meats and dairy products, is one of the most potent toxins linked to several cancers in humans. By basing your diet on unrefined plant foods, you automatically reduce your exposure to the most dangerous chemicals.

The Environmental Working Group provides a list of produce called the "Dirty Dozen" (those highest in pesticides) and the "Clean Fifteen" (those lowest in pesticides). These are their most recent lists:

HIGHEST IN PESTICIDES – *Buy organic if possible*

Celery	Blueberries	Lettuce
Peaches	Nectarines (imported)	Cucumbers
Strawberries	Bell peppers	Potatoes
Apples	Spinach	Grapes

LOWEST IN PESTICIDES – *Buy either organic or conventional*

Onion	Sweet peas	Cantaloupe (domestic)
Avocado	Asparagus	Watermelon
Sweet corn	Kiwi	Grapefruit
Pineapple	Cabbage	Sweet potato
Mango	Eggplant	Mushrooms

When we buy organic, we minimize our pesticide exposure, and we also minimize the amount of pesticides that our environment is exposed to. In addition, organic produce usually has more nutrients, especially mineral and antioxidant nutrients, than conventional produce.

GET ORGANIZED!

The more thoroughly you plan your weekly schedule in advance, the easier it will be to keep to this healthy eating style. Make a weekly plan and decide:

- What dishes, soups, or dressings are you going to prepare when you cook? Plan your weekly menu and set aside some time in your schedule for food preparation. You might want to plan on cooking once during the week and then again on the weekend to adequately prepare most of the dishes you will need for the week.

- When are you going to shop? Make a list.

- What dishes are you going to make in large volume for use as leftovers or to be stored in the freezer?

- What are you going to pack to take to work or school?

If you plan out your week and design satisfying meal plans, it dramatically increases the probability that you will eat well. Cook enough to enjoy leftovers for several days. Soups can last up to five days in the refrigerator or even longer if you freeze them. Salad dressings will last three days in the refrigerator and still taste fresh. If you are cooking for a family, double the size of the recipes supplied here so they'll last for more than one meal.

It is important to stock your pantry with a good variety of healthy foods, prepare delicious recipes, and remove poor food choices from your home. Always keep a good assortment of the right foods in the house. When you leave home for work, travel, or leisure, pack food to take with you so that you are not stranded with unhealthy choices.

The first step to achieving dietary excellence, attaining ideal weight, and enjoying excellent health is getting rid of your food addictions. Addictions make attempts at dietary modification more difficult. The good news, however, is that junk food withdrawal symptoms end in a few weeks. It only takes a few seconds of decision making to say an emphatic no to the addiction and yes to your new, healthful diet-style and lifestyle. However, the ability to consistently make the right decision requires planning. You need to commit the time it takes to shop for and prepare the right foods so that you have good-tasting, nourishing choices around you at all times to minimize temptation.

Some of the recipes in this book contain
Dr. Fuhrman's Favorite Vinegars,
Dr. Fuhrman's VegiZest, and/or Dr. Fuhrman's MatoZest

My super healthful, no-salt-added soup bases and vegetable seasoning mixes add nutritional value as well as flavor to your recipes.

• **VegiZest** – a mild blend of spices and dried vegetables

• **MatoZest** – tomato-based blend with a zesty Italian flair featuring dried tomatoes, garlic, and onion

I include these premixed options, available at DrFuhrman.com, for your convenience; however, the recipes can be made without them. You may substitute balsamic vinegar, fruit-flavored vinegars, and rice or wine vinegars for my flavored vinegars. No-salt seasoning blends may be used instead of VegiZest or MatoZest, however many of the no-salt seasoning blends are high in pepper and need to be used in smaller amounts.

If you use alternate ingredients in a recipe, start with a small amount and add more according to your own taste as the intensity of spice products can differ markedly from brand to brand.

Dr. Fuhrman's Favorite Vinegars are available in eleven flavors.

OUR GUEST CHEFS

A GROUP OF MY FAVORITE NUTRITARIAN CHEFS HAVE CONTRIBUTED RECIPES TO THIS COOKBOOK

CHEF MARTIN OSWALD is the owner and executive chef of The Pyramid Bistro in Aspen, Colorado. The Pyramid Bistro is the country's first nutritarian restaurant. Chef Oswald's vision is to develop food that is delicious, nutrient-dense, creative, and sourced from local food growers.

Chef Oswald grew up and received his culinary training in Austria. He moved to New York when he was 21 and worked there for several years before taking off to San Francisco to work for famous Austrian chef Wolfgang Puck. He then migrated to Colorado and became executive chef at several well-known Aspen restaurants. He opened The Pyramid Bistro in 2010.

Chef Oswald leads cooking classes at his restaurant, where he teaches healthful cooking techniques and gives participants advice about healthy menus. He believes that the Eat to Live diet-style will become standard practice over the next 30 years, helping to eradicate obesity and other diseases related to poor diets.

CHEF JAMES C. ROHRBACHER is a self-taught vegan chef, a certified personal trainer, and USPTA tennis teaching professional.

Chef Rohrbacher worked for thirteen years as a private chef for a small company whose owner was vegan. That experience allowed him to gain invaluable knowledge working with high-quality, seasonal ingredients; cooking healthfully using little or no fat, sugar, or salt; and experimenting with high-end gourmet and molecular gastronomy. Chef Rohrbacher is also an experienced vegan baker and (nondairy) cheesemaker.

Chef Rohrbacher worked at the alternative restaurant/performance space Cafe Voltaire in Chicago, and recently staged at Alinea, voted the best restaurant in North America, 2009, by the San Pellegrino World's 50 Best Restaurants survey.

Chef Rohrbacher eats the Eat to Live way and believes that exercise is an equally important part of maintaining a healthy, happy, and disease-free life.

CHEF JACK HUNT prepares nutritarian cuisine at Google Inc.'s Nourish Café. Nourish Café is located at Google's Mountain View Campus and features innovative, flavorful, and healthful meals served free to all employees.

Chef Hunt spent part of his youth in San Mateo, California. He moved with his family to Hong Kong and then London, acquiring a taste for numerous local cuisines and flavors along the way. He graduated from San Francisco State University and the California Culinary Academy. He worked at fine restaurants in California and Georgia before arriving at the Googleplex in 2011. He has developed an enduring passion for healthful, full-flavor, seasonal cooking prepared and served according to the nutritarian philosophy.

CHEF PAUL BOGARDUS graduated from Johnson & Wales University and has worked at a number of top-rated New Jersey restaurants. These include the four-diamond Bernards Inn, where he garnered attention and praise from his fellow New Jersey chefs and critics for his expertise in the kitchen and his charitable contributions to events such as ARC fundraisers and the Dinner of Hope.

Chef Bogardus is currently the executive chef at Vita Restaurant at Dolce Hotel and Resort in Basking Ridge, New Jersey. He has utilized his progressive, neo-American style and innovative approach to create a New York City–type restaurant that features the bounty of New Jersey's local, seasonal produce, along with healthful foods from around the world. His creative energy and fastidious attention to culinary detail have been put to use in preparing nutritarian recipes for DrFuhrman.com Corporate Immersion Programs.

TALIA FUHRMAN, my oldest daughter, has a B.A. in nutritional sciences from Cornell University and is looking forward to pursuing further education in the health and wellness field. She is just as passionate about creating tasty meals as she is about the science of nutrition. She is on a mission to help people understand that eating healthfully can be fun, delicious, and easy. As a freelance nutrition journalist, she has written for numerous websites and magazines including *Vegetarian Times, VegNews, Positive Impact Magazine,* and many internet sites and blogs. Talia was taught the importance of eating healthfully before she could read or write. A health guru to her friends, Talia has always enjoyed teaching people about how to protect their health.

CHEF CHRISTINE WALTERMYER is a co-owner of the Natural Kitchen Cooking School. With more than a decade of experience in the field of natural cooking, Chef

Waltermyer is a masterful chef, teacher, and cookbook author specializing in vegan cuisines. She has written articles for *VegNews Magazine* and *Lilipoh Magazine* and has been a regularly featured television chef and a personal chef to a number of well-known celebrities. She also contributed a few of the recipes for my book *Super Immunity*.

She is a certified wellness coach and specializes in prenatal nutrition and diets for children with special needs.

RECIPES

SMOOTHIES, BLENDED SALADS, AND JUICES

Recipes recommended for aggressive weight-loss and diabetic diets and for people with metabolic syndrome are marked with 🌿.

SMOOTHIES, BLENDED SALADS, AND JUICES

This section contains some of my family's favorite refreshing and easy-to-make smoothies and blended salads. A blended salad is a mixture of raw, leafy greens and other foods blended together to make a smooth "salad" that you can drink or eat with a spoon. Blending a mixture of fruits and raw, leafy vegetables is an effective way to increase your nutrient absorption. A blender crushes the cell walls of plants more efficiently than we can by chewing. This makes it easier for our bodies to absorb the beneficial phytochemicals contained inside the plant's cells. A high-powered blender, like the Vitamix brand, is valuable for making smoothies and blended salads. It can blend nuts, seeds, dates, and other fresh and frozen fruits.

Smoothies and blended salads are great when there is just no time in your schedule to eat a salad and chew it well. They work well for breakfast because they are portable and require minimal time and effort to make.

SMOOTHIES – THE EAT TO LIVE WAY

There are infinite blending combinations. Start with some greens, like spinach, kale, or romaine. Add in some fresh or frozen fruit, such as blueberries, strawberries, oranges, banana, pineapple, or kiwi. You can also add other flavors and liquids according to your taste preferences. This chart will help you come up with new possibilities.

LIQUID [OPTIONAL]	GREENS	FRUIT [FRESH OR FROZEN]	FLAVOR/OTHER
hemp, almond, or soy milk	spinach	berries: blueberries, strawberries, raspberries	dates or other dried fruit
pomegranate juice	lettuce	oranges	flax, hemp, or chia seeds
	kale	pineapple	goji berries
vegetable juices	collard greens	banana	natural cocoa powder
flavored vinegars	celery	cherries	nuts
lemon juice	cucumbers	kiwi	avocado
	mint	mango	vanilla

The recipes that follow give you a variety of different options, but you can also make your own combinations from creamy, cold vegetable soups to pudding-like desserts.

Berry Banana Smoothie 🌿

SERVES 1

INGREDIENTS

- 1 banana
- ½ cup unsweetened soy, almond, or hemp milk
- 1 cup frozen strawberries
- 1 tablespoon ground chia seeds
- 1 cup romaine lettuce or spinach

DIRECTIONS

Add all ingredients to a high-powered blender and blend until smooth and creamy.

NOTE: Frozen blueberries, raspberries, or mixed berries may be substituted for strawberries.

PER SERVING: CALORIES 302; PROTEIN 10g; CARBOHYDRATES 55g; TOTAL FAT 7.6g; SATURATED FAT 1g; SODIUM 77mg; FIBER 14.6g; BETA-CAROTENE 2,462ug; VITAMIN C 87mg; CALCIUM 188mg; IRON 4.8mg; FOLATE 161ug; MAGNESIUM 98mg; ZINC 1.5mg; SELENIUM 8.2ug

Apple Oatberry Smoothie 🍃

SERVES 2

INGREDIENTS

. . . .

- ½ cup unsweetened soy, hemp, or almond milk
- 1 apple, cored
- 1 cup organic strawberries
- 2 tablespoons old-fashioned rolled oats
- 1 teaspoon cinnamon
- 1 tablespoon ground chia seeds
- 1 tablespoon pine nuts (see Note)
- 1 small cucumber

DIRECTIONS

. . . .

Blend all ingredients in a high-powered blender.

NOTE: Use Mediterranean pine nuts if available. See box on page 90.

. . . .

PER SERVING: CALORIES 231; PROTEIN 11g; CARBOHYDRATES 35g; TOTAL FAT 8.5g; SATURATED FAT 0.9g; SODIUM 72mg; FIBER 9.5g; BETA-CAROTENE 533ug; VITAMIN C 51mg; CALCIUM 147mg; IRON 3.8mg; FOLATE 61ug; MAGNESIUM 93mg; ZINC 1.7mg; SELENIUM 8.2ug

Super Easy Blended Salad ✎

SERVES 1

INGREDIENTS

- **8 ounces baby greens**
- **1 orange, peeled and seeded**
- **Juice of ¼ lemon**

DIRECTIONS

Blend ingredients in a high-powered blender until smooth and creamy.

PER SERVING: CALORIES 106; PROTEIN 4g; CARBOHYDRATES 24g; TOTAL FAT 0.8g; SATURATED FAT 0.1g; SODIUM 39mg; FIBER 7g; BETA-CAROTENE 316ug; VITAMIN C 96mg; CALCIUM 168mg; IRON 1.6mg; FOLATE 254ug; MAGNESIUM 54mg; ZINC 1.2mg; SELENIUM 0.7ug

Chocolate Cherry Smoothie

SERVES 2

INGREDIENTS

4 ounces baby spinach

½ cup unsweetened soy, hemp, or almond milk

½ cup pomegranate, cherry, or cherry-pomegranate juice

1 tablespoon natural cocoa powder

1 cup frozen cherries

1 banana

1 cup frozen blueberries

½ teaspoon vanilla extract

2 tablespoons ground flax seeds

DIRECTIONS

If using a regular blender, liquefy the spinach with the soy milk and juice. Add remaining ingredients and blend about 2 minutes until very smooth. If using a high-powered blender, blend all at once.

PER SERVING: CALORIES 270; PROTEIN 8g; CARBOHYDRATES 53g; TOTAL FAT 5.5g; SATURATED FAT 0.8g; SODIUM 84mg; FIBER 9.9g; BETA-CAROTENE 3,475ug; VITAMIN C 28mg; CALCIUM 119mg; IRON 3.5mg; FOLATE 147ug; MAGNESIUM 128mg; ZINC 1.2mg; SELENIUM 6.2ug

The cocoa bean contains a unique combination of phytonutrients known as flavanols. These phytonutrients have been shown to support healthy circulation and blood flow. Of all chocolate products, cocoa powder has the highest concentration of these phytonutrients and antioxidants. It contains nearly twice the amount in dark chocolate and four times that in milk chocolate, without the added fat and sugar.

To produce cocoa powder, cocoa beans are ground and then pressed to remove a portion of the fat (cocoa butter). Natural cocoa powder is made from cocoa beans that are simply roasted, while Dutch-process cocoa powder is made from cocoa beans that have been washed with a potassium solution or alkalized, to neutralize their acidity. It is best to use natural cocoa powder because Dutch processing reduces the naturally occurring antioxidant-rich flavanols in cocoa powder.

Buying fair trade cocoa is a good practice. Fair trade certification ensures that farmers receive a fair price, allows farmers to invest in beneficial farming techniques, and strictly prohibits slave and child labor.

Green Gorilla 🌿

SERVES 2

INGREDIENTS

. . . .

½ avocado

1 banana

5 ounces romaine lettuce

5 ounces baby spinach

DIRECTIONS

. . . .

In a food processor or high-powered blender, blend the avocado with the banana, then add the lettuce and spinach. Blend until smooth and creamy.

. . . .

PER SERVING: CALORIES 172; PROTEIN 5g; CARBOHYDRATES 24g; TOTAL FAT 8.3g; SATURATED FAT 1.6g; SODIUM 64mg; FIBER 8.8g; BETA-CAROTENE 6,512ug; VITAMIN C 55mg; CALCIUM 104mg; IRON 2.9mg; FOLATE 272ug; MAGNESIUM 100mg; ZINC 0.9mg; SELENIUM 1.6ug

Boston Green Smoothie 🌿

SERVES 2

INGREDIENTS

2 ounces Boston lettuce

2 cups fresh or frozen pineapple cubes

3 kiwis

½ avocado

1 banana

DIRECTIONS

Blend all ingredients in a high-powered blender until smooth and creamy.

PER SERVING: CALORIES 297; PROTEIN 6g; CARBOHYDRATES 57g; TOTAL FAT 8.8g; SATURATED FAT 1.6g; SODIUM 41mg; FIBER 12.3g; BETA-CAROTENE 2,560ug; VITAMIN C 192mg; CALCIUM 112mg; IRON 2.2mg; FOLATE 173ug; MAGNESIUM 106mg; ZINC 0.9mg; SELENIUM 1.4ug

Orange Creamsicle Blended Salad 🍃

SERVES 2

INGREDIENTS

½ cup unsweetened soy, hemp, or almond milk

3 tablespoons Dr. Fuhrman's Blood Orange Vinegar

1 large orange, peeled

6 ounces romaine lettuce

6 ounces spinach

2 teaspoons vanilla extract

10 whole raw cashews

4–5 ice cubes

DIRECTIONS

Add all ingredients to a high-powered blender and blend until smooth and creamy.

PER SERVING: CALORIES 202; PROTEIN 9g; CARBOHYDRATES 22g; TOTAL FAT 8.9g; SATURATED FAT 1.5g; SODIUM 111mg; FIBER 6.5g; BETA-CAROTENE 8,015ug; VITAMIN C 79mg; CALCIUM 169mg; IRON 5mg; FOLATE 314ug; MAGNESIUM 149mg; ZINC 1.9mg; SELENIUM 7.6ug

Purple Monster Smoothie ✤

SERVES 2

INGREDIENTS

1 banana

2 cups fresh or frozen pineapple chunks

2 cups frozen blueberries

2 heads Boston lettuce

1 tablespoon ground chia seeds

½ cup water

DIRECTIONS

Blend all ingredients in a high-powered blender until smooth. Adjust water to achieve desired consistency.

PER SERVING: CALORIES 233; PROTEIN 4g; CARBOHYDRATES 55g; TOTAL FAT 2.9g; SATURATED FAT 0.3g; SODIUM 22mg; FIBER 9.6g; BETA-CAROTENE 2,631ug; VITAMIN C 75mg; CALCIUM 67mg; IRON 1.6mg; FOLATE 70ug; MAGNESIUM 64mg; ZINC 0.6mg; SELENIUM 2.1ug

High Cruciferous Juice

SERVES 2

INGREDIENTS

- 3 medium carrots
- 3 cauliflower florets
- 1 apple, cored and cut in quarters
- 6–8 kale leaves
- ⅔ cup watercress with stems
- 2 cups broccoli with stems

DIRECTIONS

Run all ingredients through a juicer.

PER SERVING: CALORIES 64; PROTEIN 3.5g; CARBOHYDRATES 14g; TOTAL FAT 0.4g; SATURATED FAT 0g; SODIUM 61mg; FIBER 3.9g; BETA-CAROTENE 5,828ug; VITAMIN C 73mg; CALCIUM 74mg; IRON 0.8mg; FOLATE 50ug; MAGNESIUM 26mg; ZINC 0.4mg; SELENIUM 1.4ug

Immunity Power Juice

SERVES 2

INGREDIENTS

4 kale leaves

5 carrots, peeled

2 stalks bok choy

1 apple, cored and cut in quarters

1 medium beet, peeled

Squeeze of lemon

DIRECTIONS

Run all ingredients through a juicer.

PER SERVING: CALORIES 68; PROTEIN 3g; CARBOHYDRATES 16g; TOTAL FAT 0.4g; SATURATED FAT 0g; SODIUM 84mg; FIBER 4.1g; BETA-CAROTENE 7,536ug; VITAMIN C 28mg; CALCIUM 69mg; IRON 0.8mg; FOLATE 51ug; MAGNESIUM 24mg; ZINC 0.4mg; SELENIUM 0.6ug

Detox Green Tea

INGREDIENTS

- 1 bunch kale
- 2 cups romaine lettuce leaves
- 1 cucumber
- 4 leaves bok choy
- 2 cups unsweetened green tea
- 2 cups frozen raspberries
- 2 cups frozen cherries or strawberries

DIRECTIONS

Prepare a green juice by running the kale, romaine lettuce, cucumber, and bok choy through a juicer. Mix the green tea with 2 cups of the green juice. Add to a blender along with frozen raspberries and frozen cherries or strawberries and process until well blended.

PER SERVING: CALORIES 48; PROTEIN 2g; CARBOHYDRATES 11g; TOTAL FAT 0.5g; SATURATED FAT 0.1g; SODIUM 16mg; FIBER 3.8g; BETA-CAROTENE 2,153ug; VITAMIN C 51mg; CALCIUM 58mg; IRON 1.1mg; FOLATE 44ug; MAGNESIUM 26mg; ZINC 0.4mg; SELENIUM 0.7ug

Pomegranate Refresher 🌿

SERVES 2

INGREDIENTS

1 cup pomegranate juice

1 cup strawberries, frozen or fresh organic

4 kumquats or 1 tablespoon lemon juice

1 cup water

DIRECTIONS

Blend ingredients together in a high-powered blender.

PER SERVING: CALORIES 113; PROTEIN 0.3g; CARBOHYDRATES 27g; TOTAL FAT 0.1g; SATURATED FAT 0g; SODIUM 10mg; FIBER 1.6g; BETA-CAROTENE 20ug; VITAMIN C 34mg; CALCIUM 16mg; IRON 0.6mg; FOLATE 14ug; MAGNESIUM 10mg; ZINC 0.1mg; SELENIUM 0.5ug

BREAKFAST

*Recipes recommended for aggressive weight-loss
and diabetic diets and for people
with metabolic syndrome are marked with 🌿.*

BREAKFAST

My diet-style is based on three meals a day with no snacking. Get into the habit of eating breakfast every day, then you can pass up the low-nutrient-density snack foods that may come your way throughout the morning.

A healthy breakfast doesn't have to be time-consuming or complicated. Many of the recipes included here can be put together quickly or even prepared the night before. Combine fresh in-season fruits or frozen fruits with raw nuts and seeds, or have whole-grain oatmeal topped with a variety of fruits, raw nuts, seeds and cinnamon or pumpkin pie spice.

Make oatmeal using steel-cut, old-fashioned, or quick oats, not instant oats. Steel-cut oats, also called Irish or Scotch oats, are the best. They are cut, not rolled. They take the longest to cook and have a slightly chewy consistency. Old-fashioned or rolled oats have been steamed and then rolled flat. They cook more quickly than steel-cut oats. Quick oats are cut into smaller pieces that absorb water more quickly. They cook in a few minutes when added to hot water and have a mushy texture. Instant oatmeal is precooked and dried and usually contains sugar, salt, and other ingredients and less fiber.

OATMEAL COOKING CHART

To cook oatmeal, combine water and oats, bring to a boil, and cook over medium heat, stirring occasionally. Remove from heat, cover and let stand for 2 to 3 minutes. The type of oatmeal you choose will determine the cooking time.

	AMOUNT OF WATER	AMOUNT OF OATS	COOKING TIME
Steel-Cut Oats	2 cups	½ cup	20 minutes
Old-Fashioned	1 cup	½ cup	5 minutes
Quick	1 cup	½ cup	1 minute

Unhealthful eating leads to food addictions, food cravings, and overeating. Healthful eating of vegetables, fruits, beans, and whole grains leads to appetite control and satisfaction.

Blueberry Nut Oatmeal 🌿

SERVES 3

INGREDIENTS
. . . .

1¾ cups water

1 cup old-fashioned rolled oats

1 cup grated apple

2 tablespoons currants (omit for diabetic and weight-loss diets)

1 tablespoon ground flax seeds

1 cup fresh or frozen blueberries

6 pecan halves, chopped

6 walnut halves, chopped

DIRECTIONS
. . . .

In a saucepan, bring water to a boil and stir in oats, apple, currants, and flax seeds. Turn heat down and simmer for 5 minutes.

Stir in blueberries, pecans, and walnuts. Remove from heat, cover, and let sit for 2 to 3 minutes before serving.

. . . .

PER SERVING: CALORIES 224; PROTEIN 12g; CARBOHYDRATES 39g; TOTAL FAT 7g; SATURATED FAT 0.7g; SODIUM 6mg; FIBER 6.7g; BETA-CAROTENE 34ug; VITAMIN C 8mg; CALCIUM 26mg; IRON 1.9mg; FOLATE 21ug; MAGNESIUM 98mg; ZINC 1.3mg; SELENIUM 9.9ug

Overnight Oatmeal

SERVES 3

INGREDIENTS

¼ cup raisins and/or other chopped dried fruits

1 cup old-fashioned rolled oats

2 cups unsweetened soy, hemp, or almond milk

3 cups fresh chopped fruits or frozen mixed berries

DIRECTIONS

Place the dried fruit, oats, and nondairy milk in a container. Cover and refrigerate overnight to soften. In the morning, mix with fresh chopped fruit or defrosted frozen berries.

PER SERVING: CALORIES 289; PROTEIN 12g; CARBOHYDRATES 52g; TOTAL FAT 5.6g; SATURATED FAT 0.7g; SODIUM 92mg; FIBER 8.1g; BETA-CAROTENE 597ug; VITAMIN C 89mg; CALCIUM 90mg; IRON 3.5mg; FOLATE 71ug; MAGNESIUM 134mg; ZINC 1.8mg; SELENIUM 17.4ug

Quick Banana Berry Breakfast To Go 🌿

SERVES 2

INGREDIENTS

- 2 cups fresh or frozen blueberries
- 2 bananas, sliced (only use one banana for diabetic and weight-loss diets)
- ½ cup old-fashioned rolled oats
- ⅓ cup pomegranate juice
- 1–2 tablespoons chopped walnuts
- 1 tablespoon raw sunflower seeds
- 2 tablespoons dried currants (omit for diabetic and weight-loss diets)

DIRECTIONS

Combine all ingredients in a small microwave-proof bowl and heat in the microwave for 3 minutes.

NOTE: For on-the-go, combine all ingredients in a resealable container and eat later, either hot or cold.

PER SERVING: CALORIES 362; PROTEIN 6g; CARBOHYDRATES 74g; TOTAL FAT 7.5g; SATURATED FAT 0.9g; SODIUM 5mg; FIBER 10.6g; BETA-CAROTENE 80ug; VITAMIN C 15mg; CALCIUM 35mg; IRON 2.2mg; FOLATE 57ug; MAGNESIUM 119mg; ZINC 1.3mg; SELENIUM 11.1ug

Quinoa Breakfast Pudding

SERVES 4

INGREDIENTS

¾ cup quinoa

3 cups water

5 Medjool or 10 regular (Deglet Noor) dates, pitted

2 cups unsweetened soy, hemp, or almond milk

1 teaspoon vanilla

⅛ cup slivered almonds

⅛ cup coarsely ground walnuts

½ cup dried currants

1 cup finely chopped baby spinach

1 cup finely chopped kale leaves

⅛ teaspoon cinnamon

DIRECTIONS

Preheat the oven to 350°F.

Rinse quinoa and drain through a fine-screen strainer.

In a large saucepan, bring quinoa and 3 cups water to a boil. Reduce heat and simmer, uncovered, until grains are translucent and the mixture is the consistency of a thick porridge, about 20 minutes.

In a high-powered blender, blend dates, soy milk, and vanilla. Add this mixture to the cooked quinoa. Stir in the nuts, currants, spinach, and kale.

Pour the mixture into a lightly oiled 9-inch square baking pan, sprinkle with cinnamon, and bake for 30 minutes.

Serve warm or cold.

PER SERVING: CALORIES 347; PROTEIN 13g; CARBOHYDRATES 60g; TOTAL FAT 8.5g; SATURATED FAT 0.9g; SODIUM 93mg; FIBER 7.5g; BETA-CAROTENE 2,418ug; VITAMIN C 23mg; CALCIUM 138mg; IRON 5.9mg; FOLATE 65ug; MAGNESIUM 144mg; ZINC 2.1mg; SELENIUM 7.1ug

Butternut Blueberry Breakfast 🌿

SERVES 4

INGREDIENTS

- 1 small (about 1 pound) butternut squash, peeled, seeded, and chopped in ½-inch cubes (see Note)
- 2 medium apples, peeled, cored, and cut into pieces
- 1 teaspoon cinnamon
- 1 teaspoon nutmeg
- ¾ cup water
- 2 cups frozen wild blueberries
- ½ cup chopped walnuts
- ½ cup currants or raisins (reduce to ¼ cup for diabetic and weight-loss diets)

DIRECTIONS

Place squash, apples, cinnamon, nutmeg, and water in a saucepan. Bring to a boil, reduce heat, cover, and cook until tender, about 15 minutes, adding more water if needed. Mash with a potato masher, leaving the mixture chunky.

Heat frozen blueberries with walnuts and raisins and stir well.

Top mashed butternut squash with blueberry mixture.

NOTE: To save time, use precut or frozen butternut squash.

PER SERVING: CALORIES 280; PROTEIN 6g; CARBOHYDRATES 49g; TOTAL FAT 10.5g; SATURATED FAT 1.1g; SODIUM 9mg; FIBER 8g; BETA-CAROTENE 4,834ug; VITAMIN C 30mg; CALCIUM 96mg; IRON 2mg; FOLATE 54ug; MAGNESIUM 76mg; ZINC 0.7mg; SELENIUM 1ug

Slow Cooker Eggplant Breakfast 🌿

SERVES 4

INGREDIENTS

- 1 medium eggplant, cut into ½-inch cubes
- 2 cups chopped tomato
- 1½ cups cooked garbanzo beans (chickpeas), or 1 (15-ounce) can no-salt-added or low-sodium garbanzo beans
- 1 cup chopped onion
- 1 apple, cored and chopped
- 1½ cups carrot juice
- 1½ cups no-salt-added or low-sodium vegetable broth
- 6 ounces tomato paste
- 1 teaspoon cinnamon
- ½ teaspoon nutmeg

DIRECTIONS

In a 3.5-, 4-, or 5-quart crock pot, combine eggplant, tomatoes, beans, onion, and apple.

Combine carrot juice, vegetable broth, tomato paste, cinnamon, and nutmeg. Pour over vegetables.

Cover and cook on low-heat setting for 7 to 8 hours in a crock pot. This recipe can also be made on the stove top. Cook for 1 hour over low heat.

PER SERVING: CALORIES 310; PROTEIN 18g; CARBOHYDRATES 59g; TOTAL FAT 4.3g; SATURATED FAT 0.9g; CHOLESTEROL 6.3mg; SODIUM 147mg; FIBER 12.9g; BETA-CAROTENE 9,784ug; VITAMIN C 31mg; CALCIUM 111mg; IRON 4.8mg; FOLATE 180ug; MAGNESIUM 87mg; ZINC 2.5mg; SELENIUM 9.8ug

Butternut Breakfast Soup 🍃

For a quick and delicious breakfast, make this recipe the night before, refrigerate, and then reheat before serving.

SERVES 6

INGREDIENTS

4 cups frozen butternut squash

2 medium apples, peeled, seeded, and chopped

4 cups (packed) kale, tough stems and center ribs removed and leaves chopped, or frozen kale, chopped

1 cup chopped onion

2 tablespoons fruit-flavored vinegar or Dr. Fuhrman's Pomegranate Vinegar

5 cups carrot juice

½ cup unsweetened soy, almond, or hemp milk

½ cup raw cashews

¼ cup hemp seeds

1 teaspoon cinnamon

½ teaspoon nutmeg

DIRECTIONS

Place squash, apples, kale, onion, vinegar, and carrot juice in a soup pot. Bring to a boil, lower heat, cover, and simmer for 30 minutes or until the kale is very tender.

Puree half of the soup with the milk, cashews, and hemp seeds in a food processor or high-powered blender. Return blended mixture to soup pot. Add cinnamon and nutmeg.

PER SERVING: CALORIES 260; PROTEIN 8g; CARBOHYDRATES 49g; TOTAL FAT 6.6g; SATURATED FAT 1.3g; SODIUM 96mg; FIBER 6.7g; BETA-CAROTENE 26,447ug; VITAMIN C 94mg; CALCIUM 180mg; IRON 3.5mg; FOLATE 64ug; MAGNESIUM 115mg; ZINC 1.5mg; SELENIUM 4.5ug

Apple Supreme

INGREDIENTS

- 6 apples, cored, peeled, and chopped, divided
- 2 teaspoons cinnamon
- ½ cup chopped walnuts
- 3 dates, pitted
- 2 tablespoons ground flax seeds
- ¼ cup unsweetened soy, almond, or hemp milk
- ½ cup raisins
- ½ cup old-fashioned oats

DIRECTIONS

Preheat the oven to 350°F.

In a high-powered blender, combine 1 cup of the chopped apples with cinnamon, walnuts, dates, flax seeds, and soy milk. Place remaining chopped apples in a baking dish and cover with blended mixture. Add raisins and mix well. Sprinkle oats on top. Bake for 15 minutes.

PER SERVING: CALORIES 331; PROTEIN 10g; CARBOHYDRATES 58g; TOTAL FAT 11.8g; SATURATED FAT 1.2g; SODIUM 13mg; FIBER 9.1g; BETA-CAROTENE 113ug; VITAMIN C 10mg; CALCIUM 55mg; IRON 2mg; FOLATE 31ug; MAGNESIUM 80mg; ZINC 1.1mg; SELENIUM 5.6ug

Fruity Breakfast Salad 🍃

INGREDIENTS

1 head Boston lettuce, torn into pieces

1 cup thinly sliced fennel bulb

1 medium cucumber, peeled, thinly sliced in rounds, and halved

1 apple, peeled and sliced

¼ cup chopped walnuts

2 apples, peeled and cored

1 orange, juiced

¼ teaspoon cinnamon

DIRECTIONS

Combine lettuce, fennel, cucumber, apple, and walnuts.

Blend remaining apples with orange and cinnamon in a high-powered blender until smooth.

Pour blended dressing over salad and toss.

PER SERVING: CALORIES 273; PROTEIN 10g; CARBOHYDRATES 45g; TOTAL FAT 10.4g; SATURATED FAT 1g; SODIUM 48mg; FIBER 9.5g; BETA-CAROTENE 3,271ug; VITAMIN C 63mg; CALCIUM 103mg; IRON 2.1mg; FOLATE 97ug; MAGNESIUM 73mg; ZINC 1mg; SELENIUM 1.6ug

Tuscan Tofu Scramble 🌿

SERVES 2

INGREDIENTS

3 whole scallions, diced

½ cup finely chopped red bell pepper

1 medium tomato, chopped

2 cloves garlic, minced or pressed

2 cups firm tofu, drained and crumbled

No-salt seasoning blend, adjusted to taste, or 1 tablespoon Dr. Fuhrman's MatoZest

1 tablespoon nutritional yeast

5 ounces baby spinach, coarsely chopped

1 teaspoon Bragg Liquid Aminos

Freshly ground pepper to taste

DIRECTIONS

In a large skillet over medium/high heat, sauté scallions, red pepper, tomato, and garlic in ¼ cup water for 5 minutes.

Add remaining ingredients and cook for another 5 minutes.

PER SERVING: CALORIES 164; PROTEIN 12g; CARBOHYDRATES 28g; TOTAL FAT 2.7g; SATURATED FAT 0.3g; CHOLESTEROL 0.1mg; SODIUM 218mg; FIBER 5.1g; BETA-CAROTENE 5,901ug; VITAMIN C 87mg; CALCIUM 202mg; IRON 5.3mg; FOLATE 355ug; MAGNESIUM 112mg; ZINC 1.7mg; SELENIUM 14.2ug

Polenta Frittata 🌿

SERVES 6

INGREDIENTS

6 cloves garlic, minced

1 bunch kale (preferably dinosaur "lacinato," not curly) or collards

1 teaspoon oregano

No-salt Italian seasoning blend, adjusted to taste, or 1 teaspoon Dr. Fuhrman's MatoZest

1 teaspoon dry mustard

¼ teaspoon black pepper

3 tablespoons nutritional yeast

1 cup coarsely ground cornmeal (not instant)

DIRECTIONS

Water-sauté garlic over medium heat 2 to 3 minutes.

Add greens, oregano, and MatoZest or other no-salt Italian seasoning blend, and cook 5 to 10 minutes or until greens are wilted.

In a separate pot, bring 4 cups of water to a boil. Add dry mustard, pepper, and nutritional yeast, then whisk in cornmeal and continue cooking and whisking 5 more minutes. Reduce the heat to low and stir in the greens. Cook, stirring another 10 minutes (until a wooden spoon can almost stand up in the pot). Spread into a pie pan that has been wiped with a small amount of olive oil and cool for 2 hours to allow it to firm up. Reheat in the oven before serving.

PER SERVING: CALORIES 114; PROTEIN 4g; CARBOHYDRATES 23g; TOTAL FAT 0.6g; SATURATED FAT 0.1g; SODIUM 17mg; FIBER 2.8g; BETA-CAROTENE 2,212ug; VITAMIN C 29mg; CALCIUM 50mg; IRON 1.5mg; FOLATE 171ug; MAGNESIUM 27mg; ZINC 0.6mg; SELENIUM 3.3ug

AM (Avocado and Mango) Lettuce Wrap 🌿

SERVES 2

INGREDIENTS

1 ripe avocado, peeled and pitted

½ mango, diced

½ cup peeled and diced cucumber

1 tomato, diced

1 tablespoon fresh lime juice

6 leaves Boston or romaine lettuce

DIRECTIONS

Mash avocado in a small bowl. Stir in mango, cucumber, tomato, and lime juice.

Spread a dollop of avocado mixture on each lettuce leaf and roll into a wrap.

NOTE: This also works well with collard green leaves.

PER SERVING: CALORIES 281; PROTEIN 8g; CARBOHYDRATES 36g; TOTAL FAT 16g; SATURATED FAT 3.1g; SODIUM 15mg; FIBER 12.9g; BETA-CAROTENE 2,908ug; VITAMIN C 83mg; CALCIUM 58mg; IRON 1.3mg; FOLATE 162ug; MAGNESIUM 68mg; ZINC 1mg; SELENIUM 0.9ug

Antioxidant-Rich Breakfast Bars

SERVES 6

INGREDIENTS

- 1 cup cooked or canned black beans, low-sodium or no-salt-added
- 1 medium ripe banana
- 1 cup old-fashioned oats
- 1 cup frozen blueberries, thawed
- ¼ cup raisins
- ⅛ cup pomegranate juice
- 2 tablespoons finely chopped dates
- 1 tablespoon chopped walnuts
- 2 tablespoons goji berries
- 2 tablespoons raw sunflower seeds
- 2 tablespoons ground flax seeds

DIRECTIONS

Preheat the oven to 275°F.

Puree beans in a food processor or high-powered blender.

Mash banana in a large bowl. Add pureed beans and remaining ingredients and mix thoroughly.

Lightly wipe an 8-inch square baking pan with a small amount of olive oil. Spread mixture into the pan. Bake for 75 minutes. Cool on a wire rack and cut into bars.

Refrigerate any leftover bars.

PER SERVING: CALORIES 188; PROTEIN 6g; CARBOHYDRATES 35g; TOTAL FAT 3.9g; SATURATED FAT 0.4g; SODIUM 11mg; FIBER 6g; BETA-CAROTENE 13ug; VITAMIN C 10mg; CALCIUM 24mg; IRON 2.1mg; FOLATE 61ug; MAGNESIUM 83mg; ZINC 1mg; SELENIUM 6.8ug

Berry Explosion Muffins

» Talia Fuhrman

Have you ever been berry crazy? I mean crazy for berries! The health benefits of berries are enormous, and their rich color and juicy flavors are definitely worth pining for. Strawberries, blueberries, raspberries—this treat has them all.

MAKES 12 MUFFINS

INGREDIENTS

- 1 cup whole-wheat flour
- ½ cup almond flour
- 1 teaspoon baking powder
- 2 tablespoons ground chia seeds
- 1½ cups white beans or 1 (15-ounce) can no-salt-added or low-sodium white beans, drained
- 10 Medjool or 20 regular (Deglet Noor) dates, pitted
- 2 bananas
- 10 ounces frozen strawberries, thawed and divided
- 1 teaspoon vanilla extract
- 1 teaspoon almond extract
- 1 cup fresh blueberries
- 1 cup fresh raspberries

DIRECTIONS

Preheat the oven to 350°F.

In a large bowl, combine whole-wheat flour, almond flour, and baking powder. Set aside.

In a cup, mix ground chia seeds with ½ cup water and let sit until it forms a gel, about 5 minutes. In a high-powered blender, combine white beans, pitted dates, banana, half of the thawed strawberries (leaving the other half to be put in the muffins whole), chia seed gel, and vanilla and almond extracts. Once blended, combine with the dry mixture and stir thoroughly until well combined.

Drain the remaining strawberries and stir in, along with the blueberries and raspberries, so they are evenly distributed throughout.

Line a 12-cup muffin pan with cupcake papers and, using a spoon, scoop in batter. Bake for 20 to 25 minutes and serve warm.

To make cookies, drop batter by spoonfuls onto a foil-lined cookie sheet and bake for 10 minutes or until lightly browned.

PER SERVING: CALORIES 166; PROTEIN 6g; CARBOHYDRATES 38g; TOTAL FAT 1g; SATURATED FAT 0.1g; SODIUM 4mg; FIBER 6.3g; BETA-CAROTENE 35ug; VITAMIN C 15mg; CALCIUM 65mg; IRON 1.8mg; FOLATE 37ug; MAGNESIUM 54mg; ZINC 0.9mg; SELENIUM 8.1ug

Medjool dates are larger and sweeter than the more common Deglet Noor dates. They are known as the "king of dates." Substitute 2 Deglet Noor (regular) dates for 1 Medjool.

SALAD DRESSINGS

Recipes recommended for aggressive weight-loss and diabetic diets and for people with metabolic syndrome are marked with .

SALAD DRESSINGS

As I often say, "Salad is the main dish." When it comes to salads, think big and top them with the rich, delicious dressings in this cookbook.

Instead of low-nutrient, refined oils, my salad dressings and dips use real foods, such as raw almonds, sesame seeds, other nuts, seeds, and avocado as the fat sources. This high-nutrient diet is not a fat-free program. We need to eat healthful fats the way nature intended—in whole, natural foods. Nuts and seeds are ideal in salad dressings and dips; they enhance the absorption of nutrients from the green vegetables.

Using a food processor or high-powered blender, these healthful fat sources are blended together with other ingredients such as fruits, flavored vinegars, and spices to create creamy dressings and dips that you can feel good about eating. If you do not have a high-powered blender, use raw nut butters instead of whole nuts to get a smooth consistency.

SALAD DRESSINGS — THE EAT TO LIVE WAY

Use the ingredients from this chart in different combinations to create your own flavorful and healthful dressings.

FLAVOR	FAT	ACIDITY	OTHER
garlic	almonds or almond butter	balsamic vinegar	tofu
onion	cashews or cashew butter	rice or wine vinegar	soy, hemp, or almond milk
fresh/dried/frozen fruit	pine nuts	lemon juice	100% fruit or vegetable juice
Dijon mustard	pistachio or other nuts	fruit-flavored vinegar or Dr. Fuhrman's Flavored Vinegars	tomato sauce
fresh/dried herbs	sesame seeds		dates or raisins
spices (no salt)	flax, hemp, or chia seeds		
Dr. Fuhrman's MatoZest or VegiZest	avocado		

Almond Balsamic Vinaigrette 🌿

For a Walnut Vinaigrette, substitute walnuts for the almonds in this recipe.

SERVES 6

INGREDIENTS

- 6 cloves garlic, unpeeled
- ½ cup water
- ⅓ cup balsamic vinegar
- ¼ cup raw almonds or ⅛ cup raw almond butter
- ¼ cup raisins (reduce to 2 tablespoons for diabetic and weight-loss diets)
- 1 teaspoon dried oregano
- ½ teaspoon dried basil
- ½ teaspoon onion powder

DIRECTIONS

Preheat the oven to 350°F. Roast unpeeled garlic in a small baking dish for about 25 minutes or until soft. When cool, remove the skins.

Blend the roasted garlic with the remaining ingredients in a food processor or high-powered blender.

PER SERVING: CALORIES 77; PROTEIN 2g; CARBOHYDRATES 10g; TOTAL FAT 3.1g; SATURATED FAT 0.2g; SODIUM 6mg; FIBER 1g; BETA-CAROTENE 13ug; VITAMIN C 1mg; CALCIUM 26mg; IRON 0.6mg; FOLATE 3ug; MAGNESIUM 22mg; ZINC 0.2mg; SELENIUM 0.5ug

Nutritarian Caesar Dressing 🌿

>> Chef James Rohrbacher

SERVES 6

INGREDIENTS

½ cup raw cashews

6 ounces firm silken tofu

3 large cloves garlic, or to taste

2 medium celery stalks, chopped

½ cup water

¼ cup freshly squeezed lemon juice

½ teaspoon low-sodium white miso

2 teaspoons Dijon mustard

2 pitted Medjool dates or 4 Deglet Noor dates

1 teaspoon kelp granules

2 tablespoons nutritional yeast

Freshly ground pepper to taste

DIRECTIONS

Combine all ingredients in a high-powered blender and process until the mixture is the consistency of conventional Caesar dressing, adding more water or some soy milk if needed to adjust consistency. Taste and adjust seasonings and refrigerate until ready to use.

Makes about 2½ cups.

PER SERVING: CALORIES 124; PROTEIN 6g; CARBOHYDRATES 14g; TOTAL FAT 6.1g; SATURATED FAT 0.9g; SODIUM 79mg; FIBER 2.1g; BETA-CAROTENE 44ug; VITAMIN C 6mg; CALCIUM 29mg; IRON 1.8mg; FOLATE 104ug; MAGNESIUM 52mg; ZINC 1.2mg; SELENIUM 3.5ug

Banana Walnut Dressing

SERVES 2

INGREDIENTS

- 2 bananas
- 2 tablespoons walnuts
- 2 tablespoons raisins
- ¼ cup fruit-flavored vinegar or Dr. Fuhrman's Riesling Reserve Vinegar

DIRECTIONS

Blend all ingredients in a high-powered blender or food processor until smooth and creamy.

PER SERVING: CALORIES 208; PROTEIN 3g; CARBOHYDRATES 41g; TOTAL FAT 5.2g; SATURATED FAT 0.6g; SODIUM 10mg; FIBER 3.9g; BETA-CAROTENE 32ug; VITAMIN C 11mg; CALCIUM 26mg; IRON 0.9mg; FOLATE 31ug; MAGNESIUM 50mg; ZINC 0.4mg; SELENIUM 1.6ug

Blueberry Pomegranate Dressing

SERVES 4

INGREDIENTS

··

2 cups fresh or frozen blueberries, thawed

½ cup pomegranate juice

¼ cup raw cashews

¼ cup raw sunflower seeds

4 tablespoons Dr. Fuhrman's Wild Blueberry Vinegar

DIRECTIONS

··

Blend all ingredients in a high-powered blender until smooth and creamy.

··

PER SERVING: CALORIES 162; PROTEIN 4g; CARBOHYDRATES 19g; TOTAL FAT 8.9g; SATURATED FAT 1.3g; SODIUM 5mg; FIBER 3.3g; BETA-CAROTENE 24ug; VITAMIN C 6mg; CALCIUM 21mg; IRON 1.5mg; FOLATE 32ug; MAGNESIUM 59mg; ZINC 1mg; SELENIUM 6.4ug

> Research has demonstrated consistent benefits of nut consumption on coronary heart disease. Studies show that subjects consuming nuts regularly have a 35 percent reduced risk of coronary heart disease compared to those who rarely eat nuts or avoid them. Nuts reduce LDL cholesterol and contain other compounds including phytosterols that are heart healthy.

Green Velvet Dressing 🌿

SERVES 4

INGREDIENTS

- ¾ cup water
- ½ cup fresh lemon juice
- ½ cup unhulled sesame seeds
- ¼ cup chopped fresh parsley
- ¼ cup chopped fresh dill
- ¼ cup raw cashews or 2 tablespoons raw cashew butter
- No-salt seasoning blend, adjusted to taste, or 2 tablespoons Dr. Fuhrman's VegiZest
- ½ tablespoon chopped fresh tarragon
- 2 teaspoons Bragg Liquid Aminos or low-sodium soy sauce
- 2 cloves garlic, chopped

DIRECTIONS

Blend all ingredients in a high-powered blender until smooth.

PER SERVING: CALORIES 243; PROTEIN 8g; CARBOHYDRATES 16g; TOTAL FAT 18.4g; SATURATED FAT 2.8g; SODIUM 148mg; FIBER 3.4g; BETA-CAROTENE 790ug; VITAMIN C 22mg; CALCIUM 143mg; IRON 2mg; FOLATE 46ug; MAGNESIUM 57mg; ZINC 2mg; SELENIUM 1.3ug

Ginger Almond Dressing 🌿

SERVES 3

INGREDIENTS

- ½ cup raw almonds or ¼ cup raw almond butter
- ¼ cup unsweetened soy, hemp, or almond milk
- ¼ cup water
- 3 tablespoons unhulled sesame seeds
- 3 dates, pitted
- 2 cloves garlic
- ½-inch piece fresh ginger, peeled and chopped

DIRECTIONS

Blend all ingredients together in a high-powered blender until creamy. Add more water if a thinner dressing is desired.

PER SERVING: CALORIES 238; PROTEIN 8g; CARBOHYDRATES 15g; TOTAL FAT 18g; SATURATED FAT 1.7g; SODIUM 23mg; FIBER 4g; BETA-CAROTENE 75ug; VITAMIN C 1mg; CALCIUM 82mg; IRON 1.7mg; FOLATE 22ug; MAGNESIUM 86mg; ZINC 1.4mg; SELENIUM 2.4ug

Ten Thousand Island Dressing 🌿

SERVES 4

INGREDIENTS

½ cup raw cashew butter or 1 cup raw cashews

½ cup unsweetened soy, almond, or hemp milk

2 tablespoons balsamic vinegar

2 tablespoons lemon juice

1 teaspoon dried dill

1 teaspoon onion powder

½ teaspoon garlic powder

3 tablespoons tomato paste

2 dates, pitted

1 cucumber

¼ cup finely chopped onion

DIRECTIONS

In a food processor or high-powered blender, blend the cashews, milk, vinegar, lemon juice, dill, onion powder, garlic powder, tomato paste, dates, and cucumber until smooth. Transfer to a small bowl and fold in the finely chopped onion.

PER SERVING: CALORIES 158; PROTEIN 5g; CARBOHYDRATES 19g; TOTAL FAT 8.7g; SATURATED FAT 1.7g; SODIUM 119mg; FIBER 2.4g; BETA-CAROTENE 255ug; VITAMIN C 9mg; CALCIUM 42mg; IRON 2mg; FOLATE 28ug; MAGNESIUM 71mg; ZINC 1.4mg; SELENIUM 4.6ug

Creamy Roasted Garlic Dressing 🌿

SERVES 4

INGREDIENTS

. . . .

- 1 bulb garlic
- ⅔ cup unsweetened soy, almond, or hemp milk
- ½ cup raw almonds
- 2 tablespoons raw pumpkin seeds
- 1 teaspoon Dijon mustard
- 2 tablespoons nutritional yeast
- ¼ cup white wine vinegar
- ½ teaspoon chopped fresh thyme

DIRECTIONS

. . . .

Preheat oven to 350°F. Roast unpeeled bulb in a small baking dish for about 25 minutes or until soft. When cool, squeeze out the soft cooked garlic, removing and discarding the skins.

Blend the garlic with the nondairy milk, almonds, pumpkin seeds, mustard, nutritional yeast, and vinegar in a high-powered blender until creamy and smooth. Stir in thyme.

. . . .

PER SERVING: CALORIES 180; PROTEIN 9g; CARBOHYDRATES 10g; TOTAL FAT 12g; SATURATED FAT 1.2g; SODIUM 65mg; FIBER 4g; BETA-CAROTENE 160ug; VITAMIN C 3mg; CALCIUM 80mg; IRON 2.7mg; FOLATE 171ug; MAGNESIUM 94mg; ZINC 1.5mg; SELENIUM 3.7ug

Orange Peanut Dressing 🌱

SERVES 4

INGREDIENTS

- 2 oranges, peeled and seeded
- ¼ cup rice vinegar
- ⅛ cup natural peanut butter, no salt added, or ¼ cup unsalted peanuts
- ¼ cup raw cashews or ⅛ cup raw cashew butter
- 1 teaspoon Bragg Liquid Aminos or low-sodium soy sauce
- ¼-inch piece fresh ginger, peeled
- ¼ clove garlic

DIRECTIONS

Blend all ingredients in a high-powered blender until smooth.

PER SERVING: CALORIES 134; PROTEIN 4g; CARBOHYDRATES 12g; TOTAL FAT 8.1g; SATURATED FAT 1.6g; SODIUM 54mg; FIBER 2.3g; BETA-CAROTENE 47ug; VITAMIN C 35mg; CALCIUM 34mg; IRON 0.7mg; FOLATE 31ug; MAGNESIUM 41mg; ZINC 0.7mg; SELENIUM 1.7ug

Pesto Salad Dressing

SERVES 8

INGREDIENTS

1½ cups chopped avocado

5 tablespoons lemon juice

7 cloves garlic

4 cups low-sodium vegetable juice (Knudsen's Low-Sodium Very Veggie Juice Blend is a good choice)

No-salt Italian seasoning blend, adjusted to taste, or 1 tablespoon Dr. Fuhrman's MatoZest

¼ cup pine nuts

⅓ cup fresh basil leaves

DIRECTIONS

Blend all ingredients in a food processor or high-powered blender.

PER SERVING: CALORIES 135; PROTEIN 2g; CARBOHYDRATES 12g; TOTAL FAT 9.7g; SATURATED FAT 1.2g; SODIUM 89mg; FIBER 4.4g; BETA-CAROTENE 1,103ug; VITAMIN C 43mg; CALCIUM 34mg; IRON 1.3mg; FOLATE 69ug; MAGNESIUM 40mg; ZINC 0.9mg; SELENIUM 1.2ug

Pine nuts can be expensive but they have exceptional nutritional value. They are a rich source of numerous health-promoting antioxidants and phytochemicals. They contain heart-healthy fats and have also been shown to help curb and regulate appetite.
The Mediterranean pine nut has a particularly high content of quality protein. It contains 10 grams of protein per ounce compared to the 4 grams per ounce provided by other varieties of pine nuts. This feature makes them a good nutritional supplement for athletes and growing children. Most commonly available pine nuts are cone-shaped with a dark coloration at the smaller end, whereas Mediterranean pine nuts are longer and symmetrical at both ends. Enjoy pine nuts as a topping on your salad, blended in your smoothie, in a vegetable medley, or just by themselves.

Russian Fig Dressing 🌿

SERVES 2

INGREDIENTS

⅓ cup no-salt-added or low-sodium pasta sauce

⅓ cup raw almonds or 3 tablespoons raw almond butter

2 tablespoons raw sunflower seeds

3 tablespoons Dr. Fuhrman's Black Fig Vinegar

1 tablespoon raisins or dried currants

DIRECTIONS

Blend all ingredients in a food processor or high-powered blender until smooth.

NOTE: Double or triple this recipe. Leftovers may be stored and used for three days.

PER SERVING: CALORIES 227; PROTEIN 8g; CARBOHYDRATES 13g; TOTAL FAT 16.8g; SATURATED FAT 1.4g; SODIUM 17mg; FIBER 4g; BETA-CAROTENE 83ug; VITAMIN C 5mg; CALCIUM 74mg; IRON 2mg; FOLATE 31ug; MAGNESIUM 108mg; ZINC 1.3mg; SELENIUM 6.3ug

Guacamole Dressing 🌿

SERVES 4

INGREDIENTS

- 1 ripe avocado, peeled, pit removed
- 1 medium tomato, chopped
- ½ cup chopped green bell pepper
- 2 green onions, chopped
- ¼ cup chopped cilantro
- 1 clove garlic, minced
- 1 tablespoon fresh lime juice
- 1 tablespoon nutritional yeast
- ½ teaspoon chili powder
- Cayenne pepper to taste
- ¼ cup unsweetened soy, almond, or hemp milk, or as needed to adjust consistency

DIRECTIONS

Place all ingredients in a food processor or blender and process until mixture is creamy.

PER SERVING: CALORIES 102; PROTEIN 4g; CARBOHYDRATES 9g; TOTAL FAT 7.1g; SATURATED FAT 1g; SODIUM 22mg; FIBER 4.9g; BETA-CAROTENE 618ug; VITAMIN C 29mg; CALCIUM 28mg; IRON 1.3mg; FOLATE 121ug; MAGNESIUM 28mg; ZINC 0.7mg; SELENIUM 1.8ug

DIPS, CHIPS, AND SAUCES

Recipes recommended for aggressive weight-loss and diabetic diets and for people with metabolic syndrome are marked with ●.

DIPS, CHIPS, AND SAUCES

A healthful bean dip or salsa with a variety of colorful raw vegetables is a great way to start a meal. Having a salad or raw vegetables with dip at the beginning of a meal fills you up and prevents overeating. Dips are also great when you are looking for a quick and casual dish to bring to a party.

The versatile sauces in this section can be used to add flavor without the added salt and sweeteners usually found in both homemade and store-bought sauces.

HERE ARE SOME GREAT VEGETABLES TO USE FOR DIPPING:

RAW VEGETABLES

fennel
Belgian endives
cherry tomatoes
radishes
broccoli
red, orange, or yellow bell peppers
zucchini
jicama
romaine lettuce leaves
snow pea pods

COOKED VEGETABLES

green beans
mushrooms
turnips
cauliflower
asparagus

Make Your Own Salt-Free Seasoning Blend

1 teaspoon ground celery seeds

2½ teaspoons marjoram, crushed

2½ teaspoons summer savory, crushed

1½ teaspoons thyme, crushed

1½ teaspoons dried basil, crushed

1 teaspoon garlic powder

Combine ingredients and keep on hand to season all types of recipes.
You can also add onion powder, oregano, chili powder, cumin,
or other favorite herbs and seasonings.

Black Bean and Corn Salsa 🌿

SERVES 6

INGREDIENTS

- -

1½ cups cooked black beans* or 1 (15-ounce) can no-salt-added or low-sodium black beans, drained

1½ cups frozen corn, thawed

4 medium fresh tomatoes, chopped

½ medium green bell pepper, chopped

1 small onion, chopped

3 large garlic cloves, chopped

2 jalapeño peppers, seeded and chopped (add more or less to your taste preference)

¼ cup chopped cilantro

2 tablespoons fresh lime juice

½ teaspoon ground cumin

1 teaspoon garlic powder, or to taste

* Use ½ cup dried beans; see cooking instructions on page 19.

DIRECTIONS

- -

Combine beans and corn in a mixing bowl.

Place fresh tomatoes, pepper, onion, garlic, and jalapeños in a food processor and pulse until chopped into small pieces. Add to bean/corn mixture along with remaining ingredients and mix thoroughly. Serve with raw vegetables or healthy tortilla chips (see page 103).

- -

PER SERVING: CALORIES 183; PROTEIN 9g; CARBOHYDRATES 37g; TOTAL FAT 1.8g; SATURATED FAT 0.3g; SODIUM 52mg; FIBER 4.2g; BETA-CAROTENE 569ug; VITAMIN C 20mg; CALCIUM 26mg; IRON 1.9mg; FOLATE 65ug; MAGNESIUM 73mg; ZINC 1.2mg; SELENIUM 5.6ug

Fresh Tomato Salsa 🌿

SERVES 6

INGREDIENTS

....

2 fresh tomatoes, chopped

1 small red onion, minced

2 scallions, minced

1 clove garlic, minced

½ jalapeño pepper, seeded and minced

3 tablespoons chopped cilantro

3 tablespoons fresh lime or lemon juice

DIRECTIONS

....

In a mixing bowl, stir together all ingredients.

Serve immediately or refrigerate in a tightly covered container for up to 3 days.

Makes 2 cups

....

PER SERVING: CALORIES 15; PROTEIN 1g; CARBOHYDRATES 4g; TOTAL FAT 0.1g; SODIUM 4mg; FIBER 0.8g; BETA-CAROTENE 228ug; VITAMIN C 8mg; CALCIUM 12mg; IRON 0.2mg; FOLATE 12ug; MAGNESIUM 7mg; ZINC 0.1mg; SELENIUM 0.2ug

Favorite Guacamole 🌿

INGREDIENTS

- 2 medium avocados
- ¼ cup yellow onions, diced
- ⅔ cup Roma tomatoes, chopped
- 1 clove fresh garlic, minced
- 1 jalapeño pepper, minced, seeds removed
- 1 tablespoon lemon juice
- ½ teaspoon ground cumin
- ¼ cup cilantro, chopped
- Dash of black pepper

DIRECTIONS

Place all ingredients in a large bowl and mix well.

PER SERVING: CALORIES 132; PROTEIN 3g; CARBOHYDRATES 10g; TOTAL FAT 10.3g; SATURATED FAT 2g; SODIUM 6mg; FIBER 6.3g; BETA-CAROTENE 264ug; VITAMIN C 24mg; CALCIUM 19mg; IRON 0.3mg; FOLATE 43ug; MAGNESIUM 29mg; ZINC 0.5mg; SELENIUM 0.1ug

Island Black Bean Dip 🌿

>> Chef Christine Waltermyer

SERVES 5

INGREDIENTS

1½ cups cooked black beans* or 1 (15-ounce) can no-salt-added or low-sodium black beans, drained

2 teaspoons no-salt-added salsa

¼ cup scallions, minced

1½ tablespoons red wine vinegar or Dr. Fuhrman's Blood Orange Vinegar

No-salt seasoning blend, adjusted to taste, or 2 tablespoons Dr. Fuhrman's MatoZest

2 tablespoons minced red onion

½ cup finely diced mango

¼ cup diced red pepper

1 tablespoon fresh, minced cilantro, for garnish

* Use ½ cup dried beans; see cooking instructions on page 19.

DIRECTIONS

Remove ¼ cup of the black beans and set aside.

Place remaining beans in a blender or food processor. Add salsa, scallions, vinegar, and MatoZest or other no-salt seasoning blend. Puree until relatively smooth. Adjust seasonings to taste. Transfer to a bowl and add the reserved black beans, red onion, mango, and red bell pepper. Mix well and chill for 1 hour. Garnish with cilantro. Serve with raw vegetables.

Makes 2½ cups

PER SERVING: CALORIES 117; PROTEIN 7g; CARBOHYDRATES 23g; TOTAL FAT 0.5g; SATURATED FAT 0.1g; SODIUM 40mg; FIBER 6.5g; BETA-CAROTENE 926ug; VITAMIN C 22mg; CALCIUM 28mg; IRON 1.9mg; FOLATE 109ug; MAGNESIUM 51mg; ZINC 0.8mg; SELENIUM 1ug

Roasted Eggplant Hummus 🌿

SERVES 4

INGREDIENTS

1 medium eggplant, cut in half, lengthwise

1 cup cooked garbanzo beans* (chickpeas) or 1 (15-ounce) can no-salt-added or low-sodium garbanzo beans, drained

⅓ cup water

4 tablespoons unhulled raw sesame seeds

2 tablespoons fresh lemon juice

1 tablespoon dried minced onions

4 cloves garlic, finely chopped

Dash of paprika

* Use ⅓ cup dried chickpeas; see cooking instructions on page 19.

DIRECTIONS

Bake eggplant at 350°F for 45 minutes. Let cool, then remove and discard skin.

Blend all ingredients, including baked, peeled eggplant, in a food processor or high-powered blender until smooth and creamy.

Serve with assorted raw vegetables.

PER SERVING: CALORIES 164; PROTEIN 7g; CARBOHYDRATES 24g; TOTAL FAT 5.8g; SATURATED FAT 0.8g; SODIUM 9mg; FIBER 9g; BETA-CAROTENE 30ug; VITAMIN C 8mg; CALCIUM 133mg; IRON 2.9mg; FOLATE 113ug; MAGNESIUM 74mg; ZINC 1.6mg; SELENIUM 2.9ug

Tuscan White Bean Dip

SERVES 5

INGREDIENTS

1½ cups cooked great northern beans* or 1 (15-ounce) can no-salt-added or low-sodium great northern beans, drained

¼ cup pine nuts

2 cloves garlic, minced

No-salt seasoning blend, adjusted to taste, or 1½ tablespoons Dr. Fuhrman's MatoZest

1 tablespoon balsamic vinegar or Dr. Fuhrman's Black Fig Vinegar

1 tablespoon fresh, minced rosemary

¼ cup unsalted, unsulfured, dried tomatoes, soaked in lukewarm water until soft (about 1 to 2 hours), then minced

* Use ½ cup dried beans; see cooking instructions on page 19.

DIRECTIONS

Place all ingredients, except the dried tomatoes, in a high-powered blender or food processor. Process until smooth and creamy. Adjust seasonings to taste. Stir in the dried tomatoes. Chill for 1 hour before serving.

Serve topped with an extra drizzle of Dr. Fuhrman's Black Fig Vinegar and a sprinkle of pine nuts. Enjoy with raw vegetables.

Makes 2½ cups.

PER SERVING: CALORIES 127; PROTEIN 6g; CARBOHYDRATES 16g; TOTAL FAT 5.1g; SATURATED FAT 0.4g; SODIUM 71mg; FIBER 4.4g; BETA-CAROTENE 375ug; VITAMIN C 4mg; CALCIUM 45mg; IRON 2mg; FOLATE 59ug; MAGNESIUM 50mg; ZINC 1mg; SELENIUM 2.5ug

Dried or dehydrated tomatoes add flavor and nutritional value to many dishes. They may be added directly to soups and stews, or soaked in water to cover for 30 to 60 minutes. Include the soaking water in your recipes since it contains some of the nutrients from the tomatoes.
Look for unsulfured and unsalted dried tomatoes and unsulfured dried fruits. Sulfites are commonly added to these foods as a preservative and color enhancer. Some people are sensitive to sulfites and respond with adverse reactions. Sulfites have also been found to aggravate asthma in children and adults.

Mushroom Walnut Pâté 🍃

SERVES 4

INGREDIENTS

8 garlic cloves, unpeeled (1 bulb)

1 teaspoon chia seeds

1 cup walnuts

½ cup minced shallots

12 ounces mushrooms, chopped

2 tablespoons balsamic vinegar or dry sherry

1 carrot, shredded

¼ cup chopped, fresh parsley

1 tablespoon chopped, fresh thyme

½ teaspoon black pepper

DIRECTIONS

Preheat the oven to 350°F. Roast unpeeled garlic in a small baking dish for about 20 minutes or until soft. When cool, remove and discard skins.

Combine chia seeds with 1 tablespoon of water and let sit for at least 10 minutes until it forms a gel.

Toast walnuts in a dry pan, stirring constantly until lightly browned, about 3 to 4 minutes. Set aside.

Heat ⅛ cup water in a large pan and water-sauté shallots until slightly softened. Add mushrooms and cook until tender and water has evaporated. Add balsamic vinegar, using it to scrape off any bits from the bottom of pan. Add shredded carrot, parsley, thyme and black pepper and stir to combine. Continue to cook until all liquid is evaporated.

In a food processor, pulse the walnuts until finely chopped; add chia seed gel and continue to process until mixture starts to form a ball. Add mushroom mixture and roasted garlic and puree until smooth.

Pack into several lightly oiled molds or small bowls. Cover and refrigerate for 3 hours or overnight. To serve, loosen edges with a sharp knife and invert onto a plate. Serve with raw veggies.

PER SERVING: CALORIES 251; PROTEIN 8g; CARBOHYDRATES 15g; TOTAL FAT 19.9g; SATURATED FAT 1.9g; SODIUM 21mg; FIBER 4.1g; BETA-CAROTENE 1,474ug; VITAMIN C 12mg; CALCIUM 68mg; IRON 2.2mg; FOLATE 60ug; MAGNESIUM 65mg; ZINC 1.6mg; SELENIUM 10.2ug

Herbed "Goat Cheese" 🌿

>> Chef James Rohrbacher

SERVES 8

INGREDIENTS

24 ounces extra firm lite silken tofu, divided

1 cup raw cashews, soaked in water overnight

⅓ cup freshly squeezed lemon juice

1 teaspoon white miso

1 teaspoon nutritional yeast

½ teaspoon Bragg Liquid Aminos

1 shallot, minced

1 tablespoon finely chopped fresh rosemary

1 tablespoon finely chopped fresh thyme

1 tablespoon finely chopped fresh basil

½ teaspoon dried tarragon

DIRECTIONS

In a food processor, place 18 ounces of the tofu (reserve 1 cup), the cashews (drained), the lemon juice, miso, yeast, and liquid aminos and process until very smooth. Add the remaining tofu and pulse for a few seconds, leaving some texture, similar to fresh goat cheese.

Transfer the mixture to a bowl and stir in the minced shallot and herbs. Cover and place in a warm spot in your kitchen to "age," 2 to 4 hours, and then refrigerate.

Makes about 4 cups. Will keep for one week, refrigerated.

PER SERVING: CALORIES 85; PROTEIN 3g; CARBOHYDRATES 9g; TOTAL FAT 4.7g; SATURATED FAT 0.9g; SODIUM 24mg; FIBER 0.3g; BETA-CAROTENE 9ug; VITAMIN C 1mg; CALCIUM 41mg; IRON 1.2mg; FOLATE 18ug; MAGNESIUM 35mg; ZINC 0.7mg; SELENIUM 5.5ug

Pita/Tortilla Crisps

Great with pesto, guacamole, or hummus.

INGREDIENTS

100% whole-grain tortillas or pita bread

DIRECTIONS

Cut whole-grain tortillas or pitas into small triangles and heat until crisp at a low temperature (250°F) for 15 minutes. One serving is one pita or eight chips.

PER SERVING: CALORIES 65; PROTEIN 3g; CARBOHYDRATES 12g; TOTAL FAT 1g; SATURATED FAT 0.2g; SODIUM 127mg; FIBER 1.7g; CALCIUM 24mg; IRON 0.9mg; FOLATE 31ug; MAGNESIUM 14mg; ZINC 0.3mg; SELENIUM 7.7ug

Hunger is the best sauce.
You will enjoy what you eat more when you do not overeat
or snack between meals because hunger naturally sensitizes
your taste buds for you to get the most pleasure
from your next meal.

Kale Krinkle Chips

Can be eaten as a snack or used as a topping for salads or other dishes.

SERVES 4

INGREDIENTS

1 bunch kale, tough stems and center ribs removed

2 tablespoons nutritional yeast

1 teaspoon onion powder

1 teaspoon garlic powder

⅛ teaspoon chili powder

1 tablespoon raw cashew butter

¼ cup water

DIRECTIONS

Preheat the oven to 225°F.

Break each kale leaf into two pieces.

Place remaining ingredients in a large bowl and whisk together. Add kale leaves and massage the mixture into the kale. Spread the kale out on a cookie sheet without overlapping the pieces. Using parchment paper will prevent sticking and make it easier to turn the pieces over.

Bake for 45 minutes or until crispy and dry, tossing occasionally to prevent burning.

PER SERVING: CALORIES 46; PROTEIN 2g; CARBOHYDRATES 6g; TOTAL FAT 2.2g; SATURATED FAT 0.4g; SODIUM 17mg; FIBER 0.9g; BETA-CAROTENE 3,282ug; VITAMIN C 43mg; CALCIUM 52mg; IRON 0.8mg; FOLATE 14ug; MAGNESIUM 24mg; ZINC 0.4mg; SELENIUM 1.1ug

Nutritional yeast is a deactivated yeast that provides a nutty cheesy flavor. It is available in health food stores or in the health food aisle of many supermarkets. Nutritional yeast is different from brewer's yeast, which is a product of the beer-making industry and is very bitter. Choose a nutritional yeast that is not fortified with folic acid. There have been some troubling studies connecting folic acid supplementation with breast, prostate, and colorectal cancers.

Brown Cremini Gravy

SERVES 8

INGREDIENTS

- 1 medium onion, thinly sliced
- 6 cloves garlic, minced
- 1 cup sliced cremini or other mushrooms
- 3 tablespoons whole-wheat flour
- 2 teaspoons arrowroot powder or cornstarch
- 2 tablespoons nutritional yeast
- 1 tablespoon Bragg Liquid Aminos
- 2 cups water
- ½ tablespoon balsamic vinegar
- 1 tablespoon fresh thyme leaves
- ⅛ teaspoon dried sage
- ⅛ teaspoon black pepper

DIRECTIONS

Heat ⅛ cup water in a medium sauté pan, add onion, garlic, and mushrooms. Sauté until onions are soft and mushrooms have lost their water. Add the flour, arrowroot powder, nutritional yeast, and aminos. Gradually add the water, stirring constantly. While stirring, bring the gravy to a boil and allow it to thicken. Add vinegar, thyme, sage, and black pepper.

PER SERVING: CALORIES 28; PROTEIN 2g; CARBOHYDRATES 6g; TOTAL FAT 0.1g; CHOLESTEROL 0.1mg; SODIUM 99mg; FIBER 0.8g; BETA-CAROTENE 151ug; VITAMIN C 3mg; CALCIUM 11mg; IRON 0.3mg; FOLATE 6ug; MAGNESIUM 8mg; ZINC 0.2mg; SELENIUM 3.5ug

Serve hot over baked spaghetti squash or thinly sliced strands of zucchini that have been lightly boiled.

Tornado Tomato Sauce 🌿

SERVES 4

INGREDIENTS

- 1 medium red bell pepper
- 1 jalapeño pepper
- Small amount of olive oil
- 3 cups diced tomatoes, fresh or packaged in BPA-free cartons
- 4 unsulfured, unsalted dried tomatoes, soaked for 30 minutes in warm water to cover
- 1 onion, diced
- 2 cloves garlic, minced
- Freshly ground black pepper to taste
- 2 tablespoons chopped, fresh basil
- No-salt seasoning blend, adjusted to taste, or 1 tablespoon Dr. Fuhrman's MatoZest

DIRECTIONS

Preheat the broiler. Lightly rub peppers with olive oil. Place peppers on a baking sheet and place on the highest rack in the oven. Brown peppers on all sides, turning as needed. Remove from the oven and place in a tightly sealed container. When peppers are cool, cut in half, remove and discard the skins and seeds, and chop the remaining flesh.

Place the diced tomatoes and dried tomatoes along with soaking water in a blender and puree.

In a medium saucepan, sauté the onion and garlic in a few tablespoons of water until tender, about 3 minutes. Add the black pepper, basil, MatoZest or other no-salt seasoning blend, pureed tomatoes, and chopped roasted peppers. Bring to a boil, reduce heat, cover, and simmer for at least 30 minutes. Adjust seasonings to taste, adding a little more MatoZest if desired.

Makes 4 cups

PER SERVING: CALORIES 71; PROTEIN 9g; CARBOHYDRATES 16g; TOTAL FAT 0.6g; SATURATED FAT 0.1g; SODIUM 65mg; FIBER 4.1g; BETA-CAROTENE 1,806ug; VITAMIN C 71mg; CALCIUM 37mg; IRON 1.2mg; FOLATE 55ug; MAGNESIUM 36mg; ZINC 0.6mg; SELENIUM 0.5ug

Blueberry Blast Sauce 🍃

Delicious served with steamed asparagus, brussels sprouts, or cabbage.

SERVES 4

INGREDIENTS

- **2 tablespoons chopped shallots**
- **½ teaspoon chopped garlic**
- **2 cups blueberries, fresh or frozen**
- **2 tablespoons Dr. Fuhrman's Wild Blueberry Vinegar**
- **¼ teaspoon thyme**
- **½ cup chopped walnuts**

DIRECTIONS

Heat 2 tablespoons of water in a skillet and water-sauté shallots and garlic until tender. Add blueberries and cook until soft, about 4 minutes, stirring occasionally. While cooking, partially break up the blueberries with a spoon.

Stir in vinegar and thyme and simmer until mixture has a saucy consistency, about 2 minutes. Remove from heat and add chopped walnuts.

PER SERVING: CALORIES 141; PROTEIN 3g; CARBOHYDRATES 12g; TOTAL FAT 10g; SATURATED FAT 0.9g; SODIUM 2mg; FIBER 3.1g; BETA-CAROTENE 25ug; VITAMIN C 3mg; CALCIUM 25mg; IRON 0.8mg; FOLATE 22ug; MAGNESIUM 29mg; ZINC 0.5mg; SELENIUM 0.9ug

Sesame Ginger Sauce

SERVES 4

INGREDIENTS

⅔ cup water

½ cup raw tahini

2 tablespoons fresh lemon juice

1 teaspoon white miso

1 tablespoon finely grated, fresh ginger

2 dates, pitted

1 clove garlic, pressed

Pinch of hot pepper flakes

DIRECTIONS

Blend all the ingredients in a food processor or high-powered blender. Add more water if needed to achieve the desired consistency.

NOTE: Serve with steamed or water-sautéed vegetables. This sauce goes well with bok choy, asparagus, or kale.

PER SERVING: CALORIES 189; PROTEIN 6g; CARBOHYDRATES 13g; TOTAL FAT 14.4g; SATURATED FAT 2g; SODIUM 69mg; FIBER 3.3g; VITAMIN C 4mg; CALCIUM 131mg; IRON 0.9mg; FOLATE 31ug; MAGNESIUM 32mg; ZINC 1.4mg; SELENIUM 0.2ug

Miso is a traditional Japanese seasoning produced by fermenting rice, barley, and/or soybeans with salt and the fungus koji. The result is a thick paste used for sauces and spreads, vegetable dishes, and soup.
The color, taste, texture, and degree of saltiness depend upon the exact ingredients used and the duration of the fermentation process.
Miso ranges in color from white to brown. The lighter varieties are slightly less salty and mellower in flavor. Use only in small quantities.
Miso ranges in sodium from 180 to 220 mg per teaspoon.

Arugula Pesto 🌿

>> Executive Chef Martin Oswald

SERVES 6

INGREDIENTS

2 cloves garlic

½ cup walnuts

¼ cup white balsamic vinegar

½ cup water

No-salt seasoning blend, adjusted to taste, or ½ tablespoon Dr. Fuhrman's VegiZest

½ tablespoon nutritional yeast

2 cups arugula

2 cups spinach

DIRECTIONS

Add the garlic, walnuts, vinegar, water, VegiZest or other no-salt seasoning blend, and nutritional yeast to a high-powered blender and blend at high speed. Turn the blender to low speed and add the arugula and spinach and blend to a chunky consistency.

You can use this pesto as a dip or it can be used to finish soups or any of your favorite dishes.

PER SERVING: CALORIES 84; PROTEIN 2g; CARBOHYDRATES 5g; TOTAL FAT 6.4g; SATURATED FAT 0.6g; SODIUM 16mg; FIBER 1g; BETA-CAROTENE 759ug; VITAMIN C 5mg; CALCIUM 34mg; IRON 0.8mg; FOLATE 35ug; MAGNESIUM 29mg; ZINC 0.4mg; SELENIUM 0.7ug

Chef Martin Oswald's Pesto Tip:

I make large quantities of this pesto and use whatever nuts or green tops I have in the house. Beet greens, kohlrabi greens, and even carrot tops will make an excellent pesto.
To make your own, blend together your choice of greens, some vinegar, your favorite nuts, and some spice or seasoning such as garlic, nutritional yeast, or Dr. Fuhrman's VegiZest or MatoZest seasoning blends.
You can use pesto to finish soups or any of your favorite dishes.

Nutritarian Pickling Juice 🌿

» Chef James Rohrbacher

This is an all-purpose recipe for pickling juice. It works well with most vegetables and fruits and is enough to cover about ½ pound of whatever you are pickling.

SERVES 4

INGREDIENTS

2 cloves garlic, peeled and cut in half

½ teaspoon coriander seeds

1 small hot chili (jalapeño, Serrano, etc.) cut in half and seeded

⅛ teaspoon whole black peppercorns

1 bay leaf

2 cups white wine vinegar or champagne vinegar (1 cup of each works well)

1 cup dry white wine

1¼ cups water

DIRECTIONS

Place whatever vegetable or fruit you are pickling in a glass bowl with a lid, along with the halved garlic cloves, the coriander seeds, the halved chili, the peppercorns, and the bay leaf.

Put the vinegar, white wine, and water in a small saucepan, bring to a boil, and boil for 1 minute. Remove from the heat, pour over your vegetables or fruits in the glass bowl, and let cool to room temperature. Cover and refrigerate. Your pickled vegetable or fruit will be ready to eat in 48 hours. Keeps in the refrigerator for three to four weeks.

PER SERVING: CALORIES 95; CARBOHYDRATES 3g; TOTAL FAT 0.1g; SODIUM 13mg; FIBER 0.2g; BETA-CAROTENE 16ug; VITAMIN C 3mg; CALCIUM 22mg; IRON 0.8mg; FOLATE 2ug; MAGNESIUM 8mg; ZINC 0.1mg; SELENIUM 0.3ug

SALADS

Recipes recommended for aggressive weight-loss and diabetic diets and for people with metabolic syndrome are marked with 🍃. To adapt other salad recipes, omit dried fruit from salad (not dressing) ingredients.

SALADS

There is an infinite variety of salads, from a simple arrangement of leaf lettuces to intricate 5-star restaurant creations. You will find the whole range in this chapter. Leafy greens, other vegetables, fruits, beans, nuts, and seeds all come together to provide nourishing first course and main meal options. Don't forget to add shredded kale, cabbage bok choy, onion, fennel, carrots, and beets to your salad, and lots of fresh tomato.

GUIDE TO SALAD GREENS

ARUGULA (ROCKET)

This lettuce has long, spiked, dark green leaves and a peppery flavor. Arugula is cruciferous, so it is a winner in terms of nutrient density. It is very popular in Mediterranean cuisine. Use it alone to stand up to tangy dressings and bold flavors, or mix with other lettuces as an accent note.

BOSTON AND BIBB

These delicate lettuces are types of butterhead lettuce and grow in loose, pale green heads. Bibb lettuce tends to be smaller and darker with a sweeter taste. Their cup-shaped leaves make pretty beds for bean, quinoa, or other salads. They are also great as an alternative to tortillas when making wraps. They require gentle handling and have a short shelf life.

CHICORY AND FRISÉE (CURLY ENDIVE)

Though the names chicory and frisée are sometimes used interchangeably, frisée generally refers to a cross between chicory and green leaf lettuce that is less bitter than chicory. Chicory has slender, spiky leaves with a bitter, peppery taste. Frisée has attractive, loose, feathery, yellow-white to green fronds.

ENDIVE

Endive is characterized by a unique, oval shape with very pale green tips. The taste is bitter and is commonly used in mixed salads. Individual leaves can be used as scoops for appetizers.

ESCAROLE

These broad, curly leaves are slightly bitter. Young leaves are great for salads, but more mature leaves are typically used for wilting into soups or stews. In Italian cuisine, it is frequently paired with beans.

ICEBERG

Although iceberg is the bestselling lettuce in America, it has the lowest nutrient density of all the lettuces. It is crunchy, but has little flavor. Look for green heads that are tightly packed and feel heavy for their size.

MÂCHE (LAMB'S LETTUCE OR CORN SALAD)

Mâche comes in little rosettes of dark green leaves attached in groups of four or five at the roots. It has a bit more body than many lettuces and mixes well with other vegetables. When cleaning, pay attention to the nub of roots holding each rosette together since dirt may accumulate there.

MESCLUN

This term refers to any mix of loose, tender, baby lettuce leaves. Long common in France, mesclun was introduced in the United States just a few decades ago and can now be found sold in bulk or in prepackaged bags. The mix varies according to season and grower but typically contains loose-leaved lettuces, frisée, and radicchio.

OAK LEAF

This variety comes in both red and green and grows as individual-lobed, soft, and ruffly leaves. The taste is sweet and mild, comparable to Boston lettuce.

RADICCHIO

Radicchio has deep red-purple leaves with bright white ribs. It grows in either tight, cabbage-like heads or compact, elongated ones with tapered leaves and a white bulb-like base. Browning at the base is normal, but avoid spongy heads. Whole leaves can be used to hold dip or salads. Radicchio also holds up well to cooking.

RED LEAF AND GREEN LEAF

These loose-leaved lettuces grow in large, open heads with many ruffly, deeply colored leaves and crisp stems. Look for crisp leaves with no brown edges. Leaf lettuces have more flavor than head lettuces, and red leaf adds a bold splash of color to a salad.

ROMAINE

This crisp, slightly bitter lettuce has elongated, narrow leaves that have a prominent rib that gives a good crunch. Look for dark green outer leaves that lighten toward the center. It is the go-to lettuce for Caesar salads and works well in all types of salad recipes. It keeps well in the refrigerator for a week or longer.

WATERCRESS

This cruciferous, leafy lettuce is the top scorer in terms of nutrient density. It has a bright, peppery flavor and works well in salads as well as lightly cooked or "wilted" preparations, especially Asian soups and stir-fries. Use cress as soon as possible, removing any yellowed or wilted leaves.

For an added flavor boost, I like to add unsulfured, unsalted dried tomatoes to my salads. Just soak the dried tomatoes in hot water for 30 minutes, drain, and slice. If desired, add the soaking water to a salad dressing or soup recipe.

Mixed Greens and Strawberry Salad 🌱

SERVES 3

INGREDIENTS

FOR THE DRESSING:

¼ cup raw cashews or 2 tablespoons raw cashew butter

⅓ cup unsweetened soy, hemp, or almond milk

1 apple, peeled and sliced

2 tablespoons dried currants or raisins

FOR THE SALAD:

1 head (about 6 cups) romaine lettuce

1 head iceberg lettuce

5 ounces (about 5 cups) organic baby spinach

1 (12-ounce) bag frozen strawberries, defrosted and sliced in half

DIRECTIONS

To make dressing, blend cashews or cashew butter with soy milk and apple in a high-powered blender until smooth. Add the currants and blend well.

Place the lettuce and spinach leaves on a plate and lay the strawberries on top. Pour the juice from the strawberries over the greens.

Drizzle dressing over the greens and berries.

PER SERVING: CALORIES 285; PROTEIN 11g; CARBOHYDRATES 47g; TOTAL FAT 9.8g; SATURATED FAT 1.8g; SODIUM 99mg; FIBER 12g; BETA-CAROTENE 10,056ug; VITAMIN C 134mg; CALCIUM 188mg; IRON 6.7mg; FOLATE 416ug; MAGNESIUM 160mg; ZINC 2.2mg; SELENIUM 6.6ug

Shredded Brussels Sprouts Salad 🌿

SERVES 4

INGREDIENTS

- **2 cloves garlic, chopped**
- **¾ pound brussels sprouts, cut into ⅛-inch ribbons**
- **¼ cup toasted walnuts, chopped (see Note)**
- **2 tablespoons raisins or currants**
- **1 tablespoon nutritional yeast**
- **Freshly ground black pepper**

DIRECTIONS

Heat 2 tablespoons water in a large skillet and sauté garlic for 1 minute. Add shredded brussels sprouts and cook for 2 to 3 minutes, until warm and slightly wilted. Add a small amount of additional water if needed to prevent from sticking.

Remove from the heat and toss with chopped toasted walnuts, raisins, and nutritional yeast. Season with black pepper.

NOTE: Toast walnuts in a small skillet over medium heat for 2 to 3 minutes until lightly toasted.

PER SERVING: CALORIES 108; PROTEIN 5g; CARBOHYDRATES 14g; TOTAL FAT 5.2g; SATURATED FAT 0.5g; SODIUM 24mg; FIBER 4.7g; BETA-CAROTENE 386ug; VITAMIN C 73mg; CALCIUM 52mg; IRON 2.1mg; FOLATE 130ug; MAGNESIUM 36mg; ZINC 0.8mg; SELENIUM 2.7ug

Apple Bok Choy Salad 🌿

SERVES 4

INGREDIENTS
. . . .

6 cups finely chopped bok choy

1 large apple, shredded

1 large carrot, shredded

½ cup chopped red onion

½ cup unsweetened soy, hemp, or almond milk

½ cup raw cashews or ¼ cup raw cashew butter

¼ cup balsamic vinegar

¼ cup raisins

1 teaspoon Dijon mustard

DIRECTIONS
. . . .

Combine bok choy, apple, carrot, and chopped onion in a large bowl.

Blend soy milk, cashews, vinegar, raisins, and mustard in a food processor or high-powered blender. Add desired amount to chopped vegetables.

. . . .

PER SERVING: CALORIES 202; PROTEIN 7g; CARBOHYDRATES 26g; TOTAL FAT 8.9g; SATURATED FAT 1.7g; SODIUM 89mg; FIBER 4g; BETA-CAROTENE 1,383ug; VITAMIN C 20mg; CALCIUM 90mg; IRON 2.3mg; FOLATE 55ug; MAGNESIUM 74mg; ZINC 1.4mg; SELENIUM 4.2ug

Spiced Pumpkin Seed Cabbage Salad 🌿

SERVES 4

INGREDIENTS

FOR THE DRESSING:

⅓ cup unsweetened soy, hemp, or almond milk

1 apple, peeled and sliced

⅓ cup raw cashews

2 tablespoons flavored vinegar or Dr. Fuhrman's Spicy Pecan Vinegar

1 tablespoon dried currants

1 tablespoon unhulled raw sesame seeds

FOR THE SALAD:

2 cups grated green cabbage

1 cup grated red cabbage

1 cup grated savoy cabbage

1 carrot, peeled and grated

1 red bell pepper, thinly sliced

¼ cup dried currants (omit for diabetic and weight-loss diets)

4 tablespoons roasted, spiced pumpkin seeds (see Note)

2 tablespoons raw sunflower seeds

1 tablespoon unhulled sesame seeds

1 apple, shredded

¼ cup chopped parsley

DIRECTIONS

In a high-powered blender, blend dressing ingredients until smooth and creamy.

Mix salad ingredients together in a large bowl. Toss with salad dressing. If desired, let marinate overnight in the refrigerator for a softer and more flavorful dish.

NOTE: To make roasted, spiced pumpkin seeds, combine 2 cups raw pumpkin seeds, 3 tablespoons cashew butter, ½ tablespoon apple cider vinegar, 1 tablespoon tomato sauce, and a pinch each of chipotle powder, cayenne pepper, cinnamon, and cumin. Bake for 4 hours at 125°F. Save extra roasted spiced pumpkin seeds for another use.

PER SERVING: CALORIES 313; PROTEIN 14g; CARBOHYDRATES 36g; TOTAL FAT 16.5g; SATURATED FAT 2.8g; SODIUM 51mg; FIBER 7.8g; BETA-CAROTENE 2,308ug; VITAMIN C 80mg; CALCIUM 128mg; IRON 5.3mg; FOLATE 96ug; MAGNESIUM 172mg; ZINC 2.7mg; SELENIUM 6.5ug

Orange Sesame Micro Salad

SERVES 2

INGREDIENTS

½ fennel bulb, trimmed

1 carrot, peeled

1 celery stalk

½ small head cabbage

¼ medium red onion

½ small head cauliflower

1 (¾-inch) piece daikon radish, if desired for a more spicy salad

1 orange, juiced

1 orange, peeled and diced

1 tablespoon fresh lemon juice

¼ cup lightly toasted unhulled sesame seeds

DIRECTIONS

Cut vegetables into large pieces. Using the S-blade on a food processor, fill the processor bowl to no more than three-quarters full.

Process until the vegetables are the size of large confetti, pulsing several times. Work in batches if necessary.

Combine orange juice, diced orange, lemon juice, and sesame seeds and mix with chopped vegetables.

Raw broccoli stalks, green cabbage, beets, bell peppers, and turnips may also be used.

NOTE: Portion into containers and use for lunch. Salad will keep for several days. For something different, heat a portion in the microwave for a minute.

PER SERVING: CALORIES 311; PROTEIN 15g; CARBOHYDRATES 52g; TOTAL FAT 9.8g; SATURATED FAT 1.4g; SODIUM 174mg; FIBER 17.8g; BETA-CAROTENE 2,761ug; VITAMIN C 257mg; CALCIUM 396mg; IRON 5.4mg; FOLATE 302ug; MAGNESIUM 152mg; ZINC 2.7mg; SELENIUM 3.9ug

Onions offer protection against diabetes, heart disease, and cancer. They can even lower cholesterol. Their powers are enhanced when eaten raw. Chop onions, scallions, and shallots finely and use them on your salads.

Super Slaw 🌿

SERVES 3

INGREDIENTS

FOR THE DRESSING:

½ cup soft tofu

¼ cup soy, almond, or hemp milk

1 tablespoon rice vinegar or Dr. Fuhrman's Riesling Reserve Vinegar

1 tablespoon rice vinegar or Dr. Fuhrman's Spicy Pecan Vinegar

3 dates, pitted

2 teaspoons fresh lemon juice

¼ cup chopped pecans, lightly toasted

FOR THE SLAW:

2 cups shredded apples

1 cup shredded raw cabbage

1 cup shredded raw beets

1 cup shredded raw carrots

½ cup raisins or dried currants (reduce to ¼ cup for diabetic or weight-loss diets)

DIRECTIONS

Blend dressing ingredients in a high-powered blender. Combine slaw ingredients and toss with dressing. Top with toasted pecans.

PER SERVING: CALORIES 277; PROTEIN 6g; CARBOHYDRATES 52g; TOTAL FAT 7.7g; SATURATED FAT 0.7g; SODIUM 83mg; FIBER 7.3g; BETA-CAROTENE 3,153ug; VITAMIN C 19mg; CALCIUM 80mg; IRON 2mg; FOLATE 82ug; MAGNESIUM 56mg; ZINC 1mg; SELENIUM 4.3ug

Dijon Vinaigrette Asparagus 🌿

SERVES 4

INGREDIENTS

2 pounds asparagus, tough ends removed

½ cup water

¼ cup balsamic vinegar

¼ cup walnuts

½ cup raisins (reduce to ¼ cup for diabetic and weight-loss diets)

1 teaspoon Dijon mustard

2 cloves garlic, pressed

2 tablespoons chopped red onion

2 tablespoons pine nuts

DIRECTIONS

Place asparagus in a large skillet and add ½ inch of water. Bring to a boil. Reduce heat. Cover and simmer for 3 to 5 minutes until crisp-tender.

Drain asparagus and arrange in a shallow dish. Combine water, vinegar, walnuts, raisins, mustard, and garlic in a food processor or high-powered blender and process until smooth. Stir in red onion and pour over asparagus. Let stand at room temperature for 1 to 2 hours before serving.

Sprinkle with pine nuts before serving.

PER SERVING: CALORIES 207; PROTEIN 7g; CARBOHYDRATES 28g; TOTAL FAT 8.1g; SATURATED FAT 0.8g; SODIUM 42mg; FIBER 6.2g; BETA-CAROTENE 1,020ug; VITAMIN C 14mg; CALCIUM 80mg; IRON 5.8mg; FOLATE 128ug; MAGNESIUM 63mg; ZINC 1.8mg; SELENIUM 5.9ug

Select asparagus spears that are bright green, straight, firm, and brittle. Choose stalks with tight, compact, pointed tips. Open, wilted, or shriveled tips indicate stalks past their prime that will be tough and stringy.

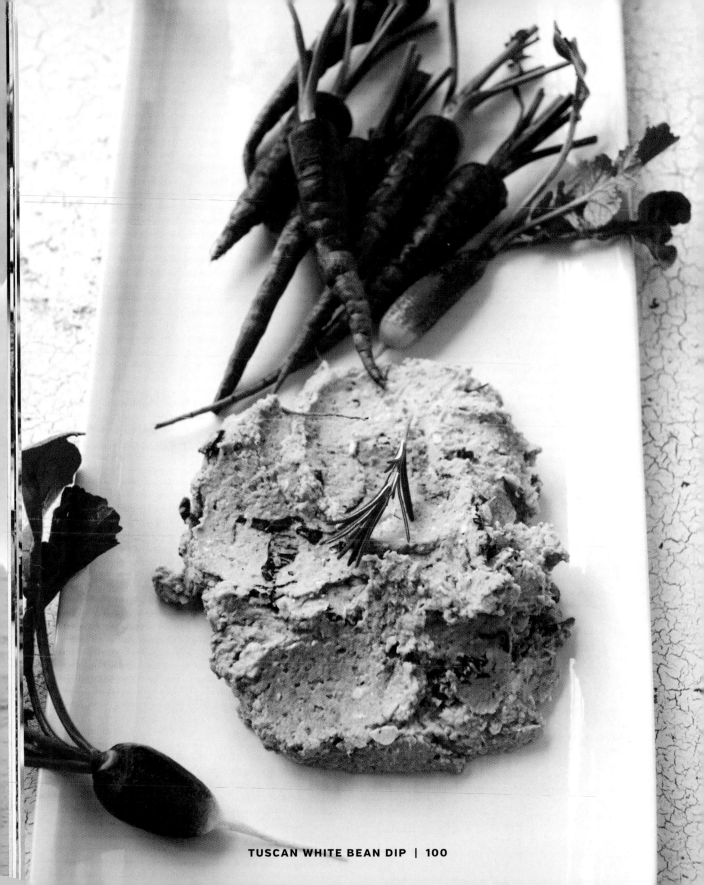

TUSCAN WHITE BEAN DIP | 100

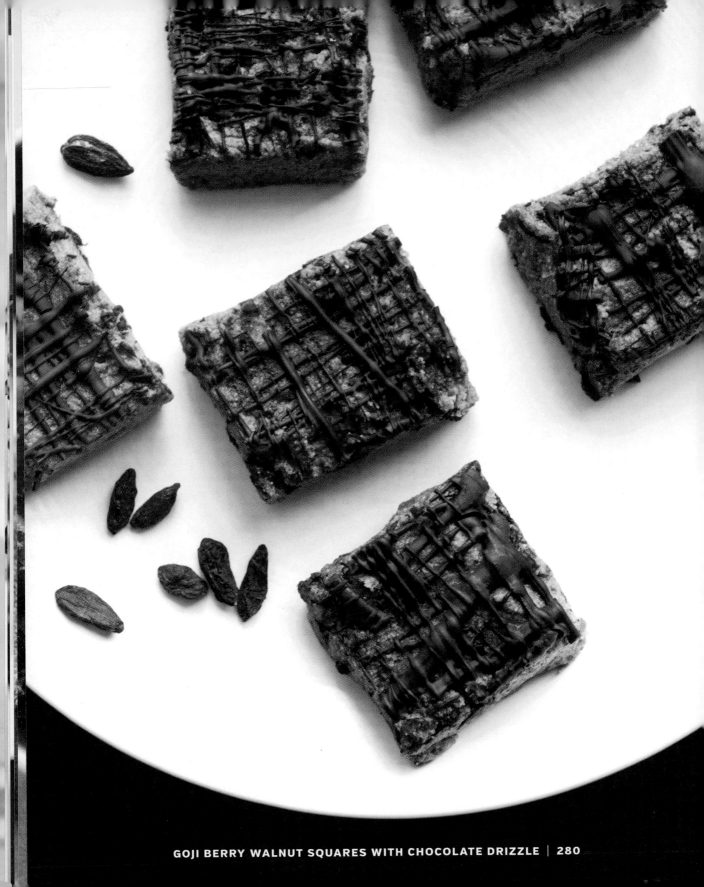

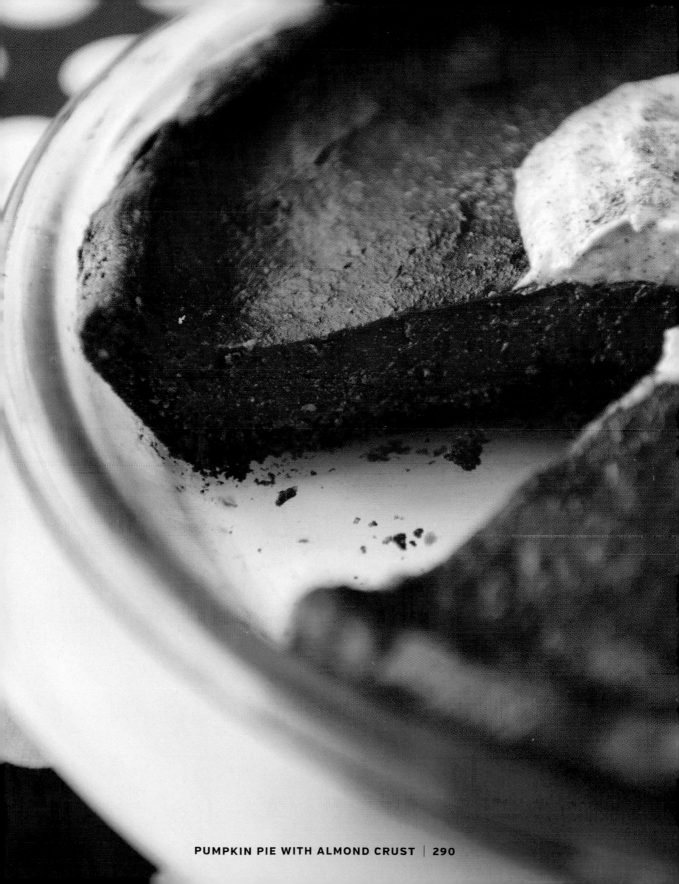

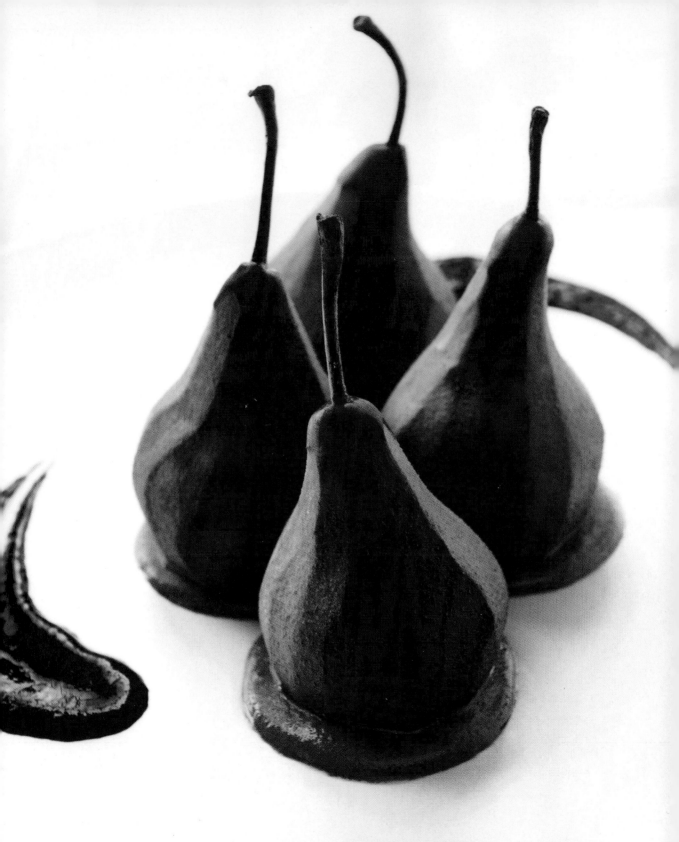

Marinated Mushroom Salad 🌿

SERVES 4

INGREDIENTS

2 pounds mushrooms, sliced

½ cup water

¼ cup balsamic vinegar

¼ cup walnuts

¼ cup raisins

1 teaspoon Dijon mustard

2 cloves garlic

2 tablespoons chopped shallot

¼ cup chopped red bell pepper

1 tablespoon coarsely chopped fresh thyme or 1 teaspoon dried thyme

5 ounces baby spinach, chopped

2 ounces arugula

DIRECTIONS

Heat a large sauté pan and sauté mushrooms for 2 to 3 minutes until slightly softened.

Combine water, vinegar, walnuts, raisins, mustard, and garlic in a food processor or high-powered blender. Mix in shallots, red bell pepper, and thyme. Combine with sautéed mushrooms and let sit for 20 minutes.

Serve on top of chopped baby spinach and arugula.

PER SERVING: CALORIES 171; PROTEIN 11g; CARBOHYDRATES 24g; TOTAL FAT 5.9g; SATURATED FAT 0.6g; SODIUM 104mg; FIBER 5g; BETA-CAROTENE 4,157ug; VITAMIN C 39mg; CALCIUM 99mg; IRON 3.7mg; FOLATE 188ug; MAGNESIUM 98mg; ZINC 1.9mg; SELENIUM 22.5ug

Salad of Roasted Beets and Asparagus with Black Cherry Vinaigrette 🌿

» Chef James Rohrbacher

SERVES 4

INGREDIENTS

½ cup fruit-flavored vinegar or Dr. Fuhrman's Black Cherry Vinegar

1 cup water

2 teaspoons arrowroot powder, dissolved in an additional ¼ cup cold water

4 medium red beets

4 cups soft-textured greens such as mâche or baby romaine, washed

20 asparagus spears, cut into 1-inch diagonal pieces and blanched in boiling water for 3 to 4 minutes

1 cup Herbed "Goat Cheese," optional (page 102)

½ cup chopped walnuts

2 tablespoons chopped fresh dill

Freshly ground black pepper to taste

DIRECTIONS

Bring the vinegar and the cup of water to a boil in a small saucepan. Once boiling, whisk in the arrowroot/cold water mixture and let boil for 2 minutes, but no longer, whisking occasionally. Remove from the heat and let vinaigrette cool to room temperature.

Cut off the tops and tails of the beets, wash thoroughly, and place in a baking dish. Add ½ inch of hot water to the baking dish, cover with foil, and roast for 1 hour at 400°F. Remove from the oven, remove the foil, and let cool to room temperature. Run the beets under cold water and rub off the skins. Cut into ¼-inch-thick round slices and toss with ¼ cup of the vinaigrette in a mixing bowl.

To assemble the salad, place 1 cup of the greens, one-quarter of the asparagus pieces, and then the beet slices on four individual plates. If desired, place a dollop of the herbed "cheese" on each beet slice. Drizzle with desired amount of black cherry vinaigrette. Sprinkle with the walnuts, dill, and freshly ground black pepper.

PER SERVING: CALORIES 236; PROTEIN 11g; CARBOHYDRATES 20g; TOTAL FAT 14g; SATURATED FAT 1.7g; CHOLESTEROL 0mg; SODIUM 142mg; FIBER 6g; BETA-CAROTENE 428ug; VITAMIN C 15mg; CALCIUM 97mg; IRON 4.3mg; FOLATE 189ug; MAGNESIUM 93mg; ZINC 2mg; SELENIUM 4.9ug (includes optional Herbed "Goat Cheese")

Quinoa Mango Salad 🌿

SERVES 4

INGREDIENTS

- 1 cup dry quinoa
- 1 cucumber, chopped
- 1 ripe mango, peeled and diced, or 2 fresh peaches, pitted and chopped
- 2 pints cherry or grape tomatoes, halved
- ¼ cup fresh basil leaves, finely chopped
- 2 tablespoons balsamic vinegar
- 1½ cups cooked garbanzo beans (chickpeas) or 1 (15-ounce) can low-sodium or no-salt-added garbanzo beans, drained
- 5 ounces mixed baby greens

DIRECTIONS

Place quinoa in a fine-mesh sieve and rinse under cold water for a few seconds.

In a saucepan, bring 2 cups water to a boil. Add quinoa and turn down the heat to low. Cover and simmer gently until all the liquid is absorbed, about 15 minutes.

In a large bowl, combine cooked quinoa, cucumber, mango, tomatoes, basil, vinegar, and chickpeas.

Serve on a bed of mixed greens.

PER SERVING: CALORIES 335; PROTEIN 15g; CARBOHYDRATES 65g; TOTAL FAT 3.3g; SATURATED FAT 0.4g; SODIUM 39mg; FIBER 10.6g; BETA-CAROTENE 596ug; VITAMIN C 31mg; CALCIUM 173mg; IRON 7.7mg; FOLATE 210ug; MAGNESIUM 175mg; ZINC 3.2mg; SELENIUM 1.4ug

Three Bean Mango Salad 🌿

SERVES 6

INGREDIENTS

1½ cups cooked cannellini beans or 1 (15-ounce) can no-salt-added or low-sodium cannellini beans, drained and rinsed

1½ cups cooked kidney beans or 1 (15-ounce) can no-salt-added or low-sodium kidney beans, drained

1½ cups cooked chickpeas (garbanzo beans) or 1 (15-ounce) can no-salt-added or low-sodium chickpeas, drained

2 mangoes, peeled, pitted, and cubed

½ red onion, finely chopped

½ red bell pepper, chopped

½ cup finely chopped flat leaf parsley

½ cup water

⅓ cup cider vinegar

¼ cup raw almonds or ⅛ cup raw almond butter

¼ cup raisins

2 teaspoons whole grain mustard

½ teaspoon dried oregano

10 ounces mixed greens

DIRECTIONS

In a large bowl, mix the beans, mangoes, onion, bell pepper, and parsley.

Blend water, vinegar, almonds, raisins, mustard, and oregano in a high-powered blender until smooth. Add dressing to beans and toss to coat.

Chill beans in the refrigerator for several hours, to allow beans to soak up the flavor of the dressing.

Serve on top of mixed greens.

PER SERVING: CALORIES 307; PROTEIN 15g; CARBOHYDRATES 55g; TOTAL FAT 5g; SATURATED FAT 0.5g; SODIUM 44mg; FIBER 12.5g; BETA-CAROTENE 780ug; VITAMIN C 45mg; CALCIUM 136mg; IRON 5.1mg; FOLATE 235ug; MAGNESIUM 106mg; ZINC 2.3mg; SELENIUM 3.9ug

Warm Braised Belgian Endive Salad with Raspberry Vinaigrette 🍃

» Chef James Rohrbacher

SERVES 4

INGREDIENTS

½ cup fruit-flavored vinegar or Dr. Fuhrman's Red Raspberry Vinegar

1 cup water

2 teaspoons arrowroot powder, dissolved in an additional ¼ cup cold water

⅓ cup chopped carrots

⅓ cup chopped onions

⅓ cup chopped celery

2 tablespoons white wine

8 heads Belgian endive, cut in half lengthwise

4 blood oranges or navel oranges, pith and rind removed, and cut into ¼-inch wheels

1 cup Herbed "Goat Cheese" (page 102)

½ cup chopped black walnuts (or regular walnuts)

Freshly ground black pepper

DIRECTIONS

To make the raspberry vinaigrette, bring the Red Raspberry Vinegar or other fruit-flavored vinegar and the cup of water to a boil in a small saucepan. Once boiling, whisk in the arrowroot/cold water mixture and let boil for 2 minutes, but no longer, whisking occasionally. Remove from the heat and let cool to room temperature.

In a wide-bottomed saucepan, lightly caramelize the carrots, onions, and celery in the white wine. Add the endive halves, cut side down, one-quarter of the raspberry vinaigrette, and water to cover. Cover and simmer 15 minutes or until tender. Add the orange slices to the pan, cover, and cook for 2 minutes, just to warm the orange slices. Arrange Belgian endive halves and 4 orange slices on four individual plates. Top each with a dollop of herb "cheese." Drizzle with desired amount of the raspberry vinaigrette and sprinkle with the black walnuts and freshly ground black pepper.

PER SERVING: CALORIES 386; PROTEIN 11g; CARBOHYDRATES 23g; TOTAL FAT 14g; SATURATED FAT 1.3g; SODIUM 87mg; FIBER 6.9g; BETA-CAROTENE 870ug; VITAMIN C 44mg; CALCIUM 92mg; IRON 2.1mg; FOLATE 74ug; MAGNESIUM 86mg; ZINC 1.5mg; SELENIUM 5ug

Jamaican Jerk Vegetable Salad 🌿

SERVES 4

INGREDIENTS

⅛ teaspoon dried thyme

⅛ teaspoon dried cinnamon

⅛ teaspoon ground allspice

⅛ teaspoon ground black pepper

⅛ teaspoon ground red cayenne pepper

2 cups sliced (⅛ inch thick) zucchini

1 medium onion, cut into ⅛-inch slices

1 large red bell pepper, cut into ¼-inch slices

2 large portobello mushrooms, cut into ¼-inch slices

2 tablespoons balsamic vinegar

2 mangoes, chopped, divided

10 ounces mixed baby greens

DIRECTIONS

Combine first five ingredients in a large ziplock plastic bag. Add zucchini, onion, bell pepper, mushrooms, and vinegar. Seal and shake well to coat.

Lightly oil a large nonstick skillet. Add vegetable mixture and sauté for 5 minutes or until vegetables are tender, adding a small amount of water if necessary to prevent from sticking. Add ½ cup of the chopped mango and continue cooking for another 2 minutes. Remove from heat.

Serve vegetables on a bed of mixed greens, topped with remaining chopped mango.

PER SERVING: CALORIES 118; PROTEIN 3g; CARBOHYDRATES 28g; TOTAL FAT 0.7g; SATURATED FAT 0.2g; SODIUM 24mg; FIBER 5g; BETA-CAROTENE 1,095ug; VITAMIN C 85mg; CALCIUM 68mg; IRON 1.2mg; FOLATE 118ug; MAGNESIUM 40mg; ZINC 0.7mg; SELENIUM 1.8ug

Chickpea "Tuno" Salad 🌿

>> Chef James Rohrbacher

This easy-to-make mock tuna salad is delicious and convenient to take to work placed on top of a green salad.

SERVES 5

INGREDIENTS

3 cups cooked chickpeas or 2 (15-ounce) cans no-salt-added or low-sodium chickpeas, drained

1 cup raw almonds, preferably blanched (see Note)

2 tablespoons lemon juice, or more to taste

1 teaspoon kelp granules

1 (12.3-ounce) package firm lite silken tofu

3 tablespoons white wine or champagne vinegar

½ teaspoon dry mustard powder

2 tablespoons nutritional yeast

3 teaspoons Dijon mustard

2 medium celery stalks, diced

4 green onions, minced

⅓ cup red bell pepper, minced

¾ cup frozen peas, thawed

Freshly ground black pepper

DIRECTIONS

In a food processor, pulse the chickpeas and almonds until coarsely chopped. Add the lemon juice and kelp powder and pulse a few more times. Transfer to a large mixing bowl.

Place the tofu, vinegar, dry mustard, yeast, and mustard in a high-powered blender and blend until very smooth. Add to the mixing bowl with the chickpea mixture, along with the celery, green onions, red pepper, peas, and black pepper. Mix thoroughly.

Cover and refrigerate for at least 30 minutes to let the flavors mingle before serving.

NOTE: Almonds can be blanched to remove the skins. In some recipes, you may not want the skins because they will affect the color and texture of the dish. To blanch your own almonds, place them in boiling water for 1 minute, drain, and rinse with cold water. Holding the almond between your thumb and finger, squeeze to slide the skin off.

PER SERVING: CALORIES 358; PROTEIN 19g; CARBOHYDRATES 37g; TOTAL FAT 16.2g; SATURATED FAT 1.2g; SODIUM 137mg; FIBER 13.1g; BETA-CAROTENE 465ug; VITAMIN C 20mg; CALCIUM 186mg; IRON 4.7mg; FOLATE 278ug; MAGNESIUM 122mg; ZINC 2.5mg; SELENIUM 4.2ug

Beluga Lentil Escabeche 🌿

» Executive Chef Martin Oswald

Escabeche is a dish of Spanish origin in which the food is marinated in an acidic mixture before serving.

SERVES 4

INGREDIENTS

- ½ cup water
- ½ cup white balsamic or champagne vinegar
- 1 clove garlic
- 1 tablespoon fennel seeds
- Pinch of chili flakes
- 2 parsnips, peeled and sliced very thinly
- 1 red bell pepper, seeded and sliced
- 1 cup beluga lentils, cooked
- 2 cups arugula
- 1 carrot, diced finely
- 1 tablespoon unsulfured, dried fruit, such as blueberries, cherries, or currants
- 2 tablespoons raw sunflower seeds

DIRECTIONS

Combine water, vinegar, garlic, fennel seeds, and chili flakes in a pot and bring to a boil. Take the mixture off the heat and add the thinly sliced parsnip and red bell pepper. Cool at room temperature for 1 hour, then refrigerate and cool for an additional hour.

Lay the parsnip and red peppers around a large plate and sprinkle with lentils, arugula, carrot, dried fruit, and sunflower seeds.

PER SERVING: CALORIES 154; PROTEIN 6g; CARBOHYDRATES 30g; TOTAL FAT 1.1g; SATURATED FAT 0.1g; SODIUM 31mg; FIBER 8.4g; BETA-CAROTENE 1,409ug; VITAMIN C 15mg; CALCIUM 84mg; IRON 2.8mg; FOLATE 148ug; MAGNESIUM 56mg; ZINC 1.2mg; SELENIUM 3.2ug

Wild Rodeo Salad 🌿

INGREDIENTS

6 ears of corn, husked, or 3 cups frozen corn, thawed

1½ cups cooked pinto beans* or 1 (15-ounce) can no-salt-added or low-sodium pinto beans, drained

1½ cups cooked black beans*) or 1 (15-ounce) can no-salt-added or low-sodium black beans, drained

1 red bell pepper, chopped

5 scallions, chopped

½ jalapeño pepper, seeded and chopped

2 limes, juiced

3 tablespoons rice vinegar

1 teaspoon ground cumin

1 tablespoon chili powder

2 cloves garlic, minced

1 teaspoon oregano

* Use ½ cup of each type of dried beans; see cooking instructions on page 19.

DIRECTIONS

If using fresh corn on the cob, steam for 7 minutes or until tender, drain, cool, and cut kernels off the cob.

Combine beans, corn, pepper, and scallions in a large bowl. In another bowl, combine the remaining ingredients and stir well to blend thoroughly. Pour over bean mixture.

PER SERVING: CALORIES 212; PROTEIN 11g; CARBOHYDRATES 42g; TOTAL FAT 1.9g; SATURATED FAT 0.3g; SODIUM 30mg; FIBER 11.8g; BETA-CAROTENE 615ug; VITAMIN C 42mg; CALCIUM 63mg; IRON 3mg; FOLATE 194ug; MAGNESIUM 90mg; ZINC 1.4mg; SELENIUM 4.1ug

Taco Salad with Guacamole Dressing ✐

SERVES 4

INGREDIENTS

FOR THE DRESSING:

1 ripe avocado, peeled, pit removed

1 medium tomato, chopped

½ cup chopped green bell pepper

2 green onions, chopped

¼ cup chopped cilantro

1 clove garlic, minced

1 tablespoon fresh lime juice

1 tablespoon nutritional yeast

½ teaspoon chili powder

Cayenne pepper to taste

¼ cup unsweetened soy, almond, or hemp milk, or as needed to adjust consistency

FOR THE SALAD:

2 ears of corn, husked, or 1 cup frozen corn, thawed

12 ounces romaine lettuce

1 red pepper, diced

1 green pepper, diced

½ cup diced red onion

¼ cup cilantro or parsley

1½ cups cooked black beans* or 1 (15-ounce) can low-sodium or no-salt-added black beans, drained

* Use ½ cup dried beans; see cooking instructions on page 19.

DIRECTIONS

If using fresh corn on the cob, steam for 7 minutes or until tender, drain, cool, and cut kernels off the cob.

Blend all dressing ingredients in a powerful blender until smooth.

Combine salad ingredients and toss with dressing.

NOTE: The Spiced Sweet Potato Cornbread (page 266) goes well with this salad.

PER SERVING: CALORIES 240; PROTEIN 11g; CARBOHYDRATES 38g; TOTAL FAT 7.6g; SATURATED FAT 1.1g; SODIUM 31mg; FIBER 13.2g; BETA-CAROTENE 4,213ug; VITAMIN C 118mg; CALCIUM 79mg; IRON 3.5mg; FOLATE 292ug; MAGNESIUM 91mg; ZINC 1.6mg; SELENIUM 1.8ug

Wilted Arugula Milanese 🌿

SERVES 4

INGREDIENTS

2 medium fennel bulbs, cored and cut into ¼-inch-thick slices

1 large red onion, cut into ⅛-inch-thick slices

3 cloves garlic, minced

½ cup orange juice, freshly squeezed

5 ounces arugula

¼ cup pine nuts, toasted (see Note)

DIRECTIONS

Heat ⅛ cup water in a large skillet and water-sauté the fennel and red onion until tender, about 7 to 10 minutes. Add the garlic and additional water, if needed, and cook until garlic is fragrant, about 30 seconds. Add the orange juice and stir to combine.

Place arugula in a large, shallow serving bowl. Pour the hot fennel mixture over the arugula and toss to combine and to slightly wilt the arugula.

Chop half of the toasted pine nuts and sprinkle over the arugula mixture with the remaining whole pine nuts. Serve immediately.

NOTE: Lightly toast pine nuts in a pan over medium heat for 3 minutes, shaking pan frequently. Use Mediterranean pine nuts if available. See box on page 90. Sliced almonds may be substituted.

PER SERVING: CALORIES 132; PROTEIN 4g; CARBOHYDRATES 18g; TOTAL FAT 6.4g; SATURATED FAT 0.5g; SODIUM 72mg; FIBER 5g; BETA-CAROTENE 517ug; VITAMIN C 37mg; CALCIUM 129mg; IRON 2mg; FOLATE 83ug; MAGNESIUM 65mg; ZINC 1mg; SELENIUM 1.5ug

Crazy-For-Kale Salad with Dijon Pumpkin Seed Dressing 🌿

» Talia Fuhrman

SERVES 6

INGREDIENTS

FOR THE DRESSING:

¼ cup raw pumpkin seeds

1 cup water

¼ cup lemon juice

1 tablespoon plus 1 teaspoon no-salt seasoning blend, adjusted to taste, or Dr. Fuhrman's MatoZest

2 teaspoons Dijon mustard

1 teaspoon Bragg Liquid Aminos

½ teaspoon garlic powder

4 Medjool or 8 regular (Deglet Noor) dates, pitted

FOR THE SALAD:

1 bunch kale, tough stems and center ribs removed, finely chopped

1 red bell pepper, chopped

1 medium onion, diced

1 cup fresh or frozen and thawed corn kernels

1 cup cherry tomatoes, halved

1 cucumber, chopped

½ cup pine nuts (see Note)

½ cup raisins or currants (omit for diabetic or weight-loss diets)

2 tablespoons hulled hemp seeds

DIRECTIONS

Bake pumpkin seeds at 225°F for 15 minutes or until lightly toasted. Place pumpkin seeds and remaining dressing ingredients in a high-powered blender and blend until smooth. Add more water as needed to reach desired consistency.

Place chopped kale in a large bowl and "massage" 1 cup of the dressing (or more if desired) into the chopped kale leaves. Let the kale marinate in the dressing for 10 to 15 minutes to allow the flavors of the dressing to soak into the kale leaves.

Add the remaining salad ingredients to the bowl of marinated kale and mix well.

NOTE: *Use Mediterranean pine nuts if available. See box on page 90. Sliced almonds may be substituted.*

PER SERVING: CALORIES 282; PROTEIN 8g; CARBOHYDRATES 42g; TOTAL FAT 12.6g; SATURATED FAT 1.3g; SODIUM 107mg; FIBER 6.5g; BETA-CAROTENE 2,904ug; VITAMIN C 69mg; CALCIUM 102mg; IRON 3.3mg; FOLATE 54ug; MAGNESIUM 104mg; ZINC 1.9mg; SELENIUM 1.2ug

Warm Spiced Butternut Squash Salad with Winesap Apples

>> Executive Chef Martin Oswald

SERVES 4

INGREDIENTS

FOR THE DRESSING:

1 clove garlic

1 tablespoon chopped shallots

2 tablespoons apple cider vinegar

1 tablespoon Dijon mustard

½ cup unsweetened apple juice or water

2 tablespoons raw almond butter

1 Medjool date or 2 regular dates, pitted

½ cup parsley

6 sage leaves

FOR THE BUTTERNUT SQUASH:

12 ounces butternut squash, peeled and cut into ¾-inch dice

1 tablespoon date sugar, optional

Pinch of ground cinnamon

Pinch of ground cloves

Pinch of ground allspice

Pinch of cayenne

½ cup unsweetened apple juice

FOR THE SALAD:

4 tablespoons raw pumpkin seeds

2 apples (Winesap or other local apple), diced

2 tablespoons chopped, dried apples

2 tablespoons red onions, sliced

3 cups spinach, sliced

3 cups kale, sliced very thinly

DIRECTIONS

Combine dressing ingredients in a high-powered blender. Blend at high speed until combined.

Preheat the oven to 350°F.

To roast the butternut squash, mix the squash with the date sugar, cinnamon, cloves, allspice, cayenne, and apple juice. Place the mixture in a baking pan, cover with foil, and roast until caramelized but still firm when a fork is inserted, about 15 minutes, stirring halfway through cooking time.

While the squash is roasting, combine pumpkin seeds, apples, dried apples, onions, spinach, and kale in a bowl.

Remove squash from the oven and combine with dressing. Pour over the salad, mix to combine, and serve immediately.

PER SERVING: CALORIES 271; PROTEIN 9g; CARBOHYDRATES 45g; TOTAL FAT 9.4g; SATURATED FAT 1.3g; SODIUM 147mg; FIBER 6.1g; BETA-CAROTENE 9,915ug; VITAMIN C 99mg; CALCIUM 185mg; IRON 4.6mg; FOLATE 107ug; MAGNESIUM 146mg; ZINC 1.7mg; SELENIUM 1.9ug

This salad shines with all the great produce the fall season has to offer. When cooking the butternut squash pieces, you want to lightly brown them on all sides to release their natural sugar; also as they turn color, check repeatedly for doneness by poking them with a fork or knife. A little resistance when inserting the fork will guarantee a good "bite" and lots of smiling faces. In place of butternut squash you can use sweet potatoes, parsnip, delicata squash, acorn squash, or buttercup squash.

Ginger-Poached Butternut Squash Salad with Warm Ginger Raisin Dressing 🌿

≫ Chef Jack Hunt

The leftover broth can be saved for a delicious soup the next day!

SERVES 4

INGREDIENTS

- 3 cups low-sodium or no-salt-added vegetable stock
- ½ bunch celery, washed, trimmed, and diced
- ½ yellow onion, trimmed, peeled, and diced
- 1 red Fresno chili or jalapeño
- ¼ cup finely minced ginger
- ½ large butternut squash, washed, peeled, and cut into 1-inch half-moons
- 2 tablespoons rice wine vinegar
- ¼ cup raisins or other unsulfured dried fruit
- ½ bunch dino/lacinato kale, de-stemmed, washed, and finely chopped
- 1 cup bean sprouts
- ½ pint cherry tomatoes
- 1 cup basil and mint leaves
- 2 tablespoons chopped garlic
- ¼ cup raw cashews, lightly toasted, coarsely chopped

DIRECTIONS

Place vegetable stock in a high-sided pot and add celery, onion, garlic, chili, and ginger. Bring to a boil, then reduce to a very low simmer (under 180°F). Simmer for 5 minutes, then add the butternut squash. Place a lid on the pot and poach slowly for 20 to 30 minutes. Remove squash with a slotted spoon, place on a plate, and keep warm. Reserve the broth and remaining cooked vegetables.

Pour ½ cup of the broth into a small bowl and add the rice wine vinegar and raisins to allow the raisins to plump and absorb some broth.

Place the kale, sprouts, tomatoes, herbs, and ½ cup of cooked vegetables (from the broth) into a large mixing bowl.

Puree the raisin mixture with an immersion blender or high-powered blender. Add desired amount to kale salad.

Place the salad on large plates, top with the poached squash, and garnish with cashews.

PER SERVING: CALORIES 268; PROTEIN 13g; CARBOHYDRATES 49g; TOTAL FAT 6.2g; SATURATED FAT 1.2g; SODIUM 110mg; FIBER 7.7g; BETA-CAROTENE 13,358ug; VITAMIN C 110mg; CALCIUM 227mg; IRON 4.3mg; FOLATE 129ug; MAGNESIUM 146mg; ZINC 1.6mg; SELENIUM 3.9ug

Chewing green vegetables very well releases more of their anticancer compounds. If you mix some raw cabbage, kale, arugula, or watercress in your salad and chew well, it will actually increase the nutrients released from the cooked greens you consume in the same meal.

SOUPS AND STEWS

*Recipes recommended for aggressive weight-loss
and diabetic diets and for people
with metabolic syndrome are marked with* 🌱.

SOUPS AND STEWS

Soups play a big role in my diet-style. When vegetables are simmered in soup, all the nutrients are retained in the liquid and the gentle heat prevents nutrient loss.

Soups and stews are cooked at 212°F, the boiling point of water. Cooking at this low temperature in water is healthful because cooking by-products called acrylamides are not formed. Acrylamides are compounds that can cause genetic mutations, increasing the risk of cancer. They are formed during high-temperature cooking such as frying, baking, roasting, and grilling. Steamed or boiled foods, on the other hand, do not contain these compounds.

It is easy to incorporate a variety of green leafy vegetables, mushrooms, onions, beans, and other healthy ingredients all in one pot. A big advantage to making soups and stews is that they make great leftovers. I like to make a large pot of soup for dinner and then have lunch for several days. Soups generally keep well for up to five days in the refrigerator and can be frozen in individual containers if longer storage is desired.

To make a "cream" soup, raw cashews, pine nuts, almonds, or hemp seeds can be blended into the soup to provide a creamy texture and rich flavor. In many of my recipes, a portion of the cooked soup is removed from the pot and blended with raw nuts or seeds. This blended portion is then added back to the pot. If you are allergic to nuts or seeds, you can just blend a portion of the soup without adding the nuts. It will still give you a creamy texture.

I use vegetable juices, such as carrot juice, for the base of many of my soups. For maximum flavor, use freshly juiced carrot juice. Fresh juice from organic carrots tastes the best. If you are short on time, store-bought, refrigerated, bottled carrot juice can be used. Homemade or purchased no-salt-added or low-sodium vegetable broth is also used in some soup recipes. As a general guideline, do not use a store-bought vegetable broth that has more than 200 mg of sodium per one cup serving.

SOUPS AND STEWS — THE EAT TO LIVE WAY

Once you get the general idea, you can mix and match ingredients.

Start with a base such as carrot juice, tomato juice, or low-sodium or no-salt-added prepared broth. Add some leafy greens, a member of the onion family, some flavoring like VegiZest, and any other vegetables that you have on hand. Don't forget the beans. Create all-new soups by matching up different items from the columns in the chart below.

BASE	LEAFY GREENS	ALLIUM FAMILY	OTHER VEGGIES	FLAVOR	BEANS
carrot juice	kale	onion	fresh or dried tomato	no-salt seasoning blends or Dr. Fuhrman's VegiZest or MatoZest	cannellini or other white beans
low-sodium or no-salt-added vegetable broth	spinach	leeks	mushrooms	basil, cilantro, parsley, or dill	red kidney
low-sodium tomato juice	collards or mustard greens	garlic	red or green bell pepper	thyme, oregano, rosemary, sage, or marjoram	lentils or split peas
celery juice	Swiss chard	chives	broccoli	bay leaves	black beans
low-sodium V8	bok choy	shallots	squash or sweet potato	chili powder or cumin	garbanzo beans / chickpeas
beet juice	cabbage	ginger*	carrots and celery	curry powder	pinto beans
			zucchini	lemon or lime	edamame or tofu
			parsnips	cayenne or other hot pepper flakes	

* Not in allium family

Homemade Vegetable Broth 🌿

SERVES 8

INGREDIENTS

- 2 medium onions, chopped
- 1 cup finely chopped scallions
- 4 carrots, chopped
- 2 stalks celery, chopped
- 2 cups mushrooms, chopped
- 2 medium tomatoes, chopped
- 3 cloves garlic, peeled and halved crosswise
- 3 bay leaves
- 1 cup chopped fresh dill
- ½ cup chopped fresh parsley
- 6 whole black peppercorns
- 1 teaspoon dried oregano
- 14 cups water

DIRECTIONS

Place all ingredients in a large pot and bring to a boil. Reduce heat and simmer for at least 1 hour. Skim and discard any foam from surface.

Strain the broth, discard the bay leaves, but reserve the vegetables to eat separately or puree them and use to thicken soups or sauces.

Use in soup recipes instead of store-bought vegetable broth. Can be frozen in small containers; will keep frozen up to six months.

PER SERVING: CALORIES 43; PROTEIN 3g; CARBOHYDRATES 9g; TOTAL FAT 0.3g; SATURATED FAT 0.1g; SODIUM 49mg; FIBER 2.8g; BETA-CAROTENE 3,178ug; VITAMIN C 20mg; CALCIUM 57mg; IRON 1mg; FOLATE 33ug; MAGNESIUM 23mg; ZINC 0.4mg; SELENIUM 2.7ug

Acorn Squash Stew with Brussels Sprouts 🌿

SERVES 4

INGREDIENTS

1 small onion, chopped

6 cloves garlic, minced

1 small fennel bulb, trimmed, cored, and thinly sliced

2 cups acorn squash, peeled and cut into ¾-inch pieces

8 ounces brussels sprouts, trimmed and halved

4 cups low-sodium or no-salt-added vegetable broth

2 tablespoons fresh sage, crushed

1 tablespoon fresh rosemary, crushed, or 1 teaspoon dried rosemary, crushed

1 apple, cored and coarsely chopped

6 dried, unsulfured apricots, finely chopped

1½ cups cooked red kidney beans* or 1 (15-ounce) can low-sodium or no-salt-added kidney beans, drained

1 tablespoon sherry vinegar or balsamic vinegar

Freshly ground pepper to taste

* Use ½ cup dried beans; see cooking instructions on page 19.

DIRECTIONS

Heat ⅛ cup water in a large pot, add onion and garlic, and water-sauté until tender, about 4 minutes. Add fennel, squash, brussels sprouts, broth, sage, and rosemary. Bring to boiling, reduce heat. Cover and simmer, about 10 minutes or until vegetables are nearly tender.

Add apple and apricots. Cook covered, about 5 minutes more or just until brussels sprouts are tender. Add beans and vinegar and heat through. Season with pepper.

PER SERVING: CALORIES 246; PROTEIN 15g; CARBOHYDRATES 48g; TOTAL FAT 2.3g; SATURATED FAT 0.6g; SODIUM 124mg; FIBER 11.8g; BETA-CAROTENE 532ug; VITAMIN C 69mg; CALCIUM 126mg; IRON 4.5mg; FOLATE 156ug; MAGNESIUM 86mg; ZINC 1.5mg; SELENIUM 3.4ug

Make a vegetable-bean soup on the weekend and you can use it for lunch every day for the whole week.

Black Forest Cream of Mushroom Soup 🌿

INGREDIENTS

2 pounds mixed, fresh mushrooms (button, shiitake, cremini), sliced ¼ inch thick

2 cloves garlic, minced or pressed

2 teaspoons herbes de Provence

5 cups carrot juice (5 pounds carrots, juiced)

3 cups unsweetened hemp, soy, or almond milk, divided

2 carrots, coarsely chopped

2 medium onions, chopped

¾ cup fresh or frozen corn kernels

1 cup chopped celery

3 leeks, cut in ½-inch-thick rounds

No-salt seasoning blend, adjusted to taste, or ¼ cup Dr. Fuhrman's VegiZest

¼ cup raw cashews

1 tablespoon fresh lemon juice

1 tablespoon chopped fresh thyme

2 teaspoons chopped fresh rosemary

3 cups cooked white beans* (northern, navy, cannellini) or 2 (15-ounce) cans no-salt-added or low-sodium white beans, drained

5 ounces baby spinach

¼ cup chopped fresh parsley, for garnish

* Use 1 cup dried beans; see bean cooking instructions on page 19.

DIRECTIONS

In a large soup pot, bring the carrot juice, 2½ cups of the milk, carrots, onion, corn, celery, leeks, and VegiZest or other no-salt seasoning blend to a boil. Add the mushrooms, garlic, and herbes de Provence. Reduce the heat and simmer until the vegetables are tender, about 30 minutes.

In a food processor or high-powered blender, puree the cashews and remaining ½ cup milk. Add half of the soup liquid and vegetables, the lemon juice, thyme, and rosemary. Blend until smooth and creamy.

Return the pureed soup mixture to the pot. Add the beans, spinach, and sautéed mushrooms. Heat until the spinach is wilted. Garnish with parsley.

PER SERVING: CALORIES 305; PROTEIN 18g; CARBOHYDRATES 53g; TOTAL FAT 5.1g; SATURATED FAT 0.9g; SODIUM 164mg; FIBER 11g; BETA-CAROTENE 17,408ug; VITAMIN C 36mg; CALCIUM 186mg; IRON 6mg; FOLATE 188ug; MAGNESIUM 133mg; ZINC 2.4mg; SELENIUM 19.9ug

Broccoli Mushroom Bisque 🌿

SERVES 4

INGREDIENTS

- 1 head broccoli, cut into florets
- 8 ounces mushrooms, sliced
- 3 carrots, coarsely chopped
- 1 cup coarsely chopped celery
- 1 onion, chopped
- 4 cloves garlic, minced
- 2 teaspoons Mrs. Dash no-salt seasoning blend or 2 tablespoons Dr. Fuhrman's VegiZest
- 2 cups carrot juice (2 pounds carrots, juiced)
- 4 cups water
- ½ teaspoon nutmeg
- ½ cup raw cashews
- ½ cup pine nuts (use Mediterranean pine nuts if available)

DIRECTIONS

Place all the ingredients, except the cashews and pine nuts, in a soup pot. Cover and simmer for 20 minutes or until the vegetables are just tender.

In a food processor or high-powered blender, blend two-thirds of the soup liquid and vegetables with the cashews and pine nuts until smooth and creamy. Return to the pot and reheat before serving.

PER SERVING: CALORIES 339; PROTEIN 13g; CARBOHYDRATES 37g; TOTAL FAT 19g; SATURATED FAT 2.1g; SODIUM 157mg; FIBER 7.8g; BETA-CAROTENE 15,850ug; VITAMIN C 121mg; CALCIUM 133mg; IRON 4.2mg; FOLATE 118ug; MAGNESIUM 144mg; ZINC 3.1mg; SELENIUM 12.2ug

"Cheesy" Kale Soup 🌿

SERVES 4

INGREDIENTS

½ cup yellow split peas

1 onion, chopped

1 cup mushrooms, sliced

2 cups carrot juice
(2 pounds carrots, juiced)

15 ounces no-salt-added or
low-sodium tomato sauce

1½ pounds kale, tough stems and
center ribs removed and leaves
coarsely chopped

½ cup raw cashew butter

2 tablespoons nutritional yeast

DIRECTIONS

In a pressure cooker, cover yellow split peas with about 2½ cups water and cook on
high pressure for 6 to 8 minutes.

Add remaining ingredients except cashew butter and nutritional yeast and cook on
high pressure for 1 minute. Release pressure and blend soup with cashew butter.

Sprinkle with nutritional yeast before serving.

TO MAKE WITHOUT A PRESSURE COOKER:

Precook the split peas until soft.

Combine cooked split peas with all remaining ingredients except cashew butter and
nutritional yeast. Bring to a boil, reduce heat, and simmer until kale is tender (about
15 minutes). Add water as needed to achieve desired consistency. Stir in cashew
butter. Sprinkle with nutritional yeast before serving.

PER SERVING: CALORIES 363; PROTEIN 18g; CARBOHYDRATES 58g; TOTAL FAT 9.9g; SATURATED FAT 1.8g; SODIUM 127mg;
FIBER 13g; BETA-CAROTENE 26,913ug; VITAMIN C 231mg; CALCIUM 300mg; IRON 6.3mg; FOLATE 148ug; MAGNESIUM 168mg;
ZINC 2.9mg; SELENIUM 7.5ug

Chunky Sweet Potato Stew 🌿

SERVES 2

INGREDIENTS

1 onion, thickly sliced

2 large garlic cloves, chopped

1½ cups stewed tomatoes with juice

1 large sweet potato, peeled and cut into ½-inch pieces

1 cup cooked* or canned no-salt-added or low-sodium garbanzo beans (chickpeas) or white kidney beans

¾ teaspoon dried rosemary

1 medium zucchini, cut into ½-inch-thick rounds

1 teaspoon Mrs. Dash no-salt seasoning

* Use ⅓ cup dried beans; see bean cooking instructions on page 19.

DIRECTIONS

In a sauté pan, heat 2 tablespoons water. Add the onion and water-sauté about 5 minutes, until slightly softened, separating slices into rings. Add garlic and cook 1 minute. Add water as necessary to prevent from scorching.

Mix in stewed tomatoes with juice, sweet potato, garbanzo beans, and rosemary. Bring mixture to a simmer, stirring occasionally. Cover and cook 5 minutes. Add zucchini. Cover and cook until sweet potatoes are tender, about 15 minutes, stirring occasionally. Season with Mrs. Dash.

NOTE: To make homemade stewed tomatoes: Place whole tomatoes in boiling water for 1 minute and then immediately transfer to cold water. Peel and quarter tomatoes, and place in a large saucepan. Slowly simmer over low heat for 20 to 30 minutes, stirring occasionally to prevent burning.

PER SERVING: CALORIES 253; PROTEIN 9g; CARBOHYDRATES 50g; TOTAL FAT 3.6g; SATURATED FAT 0.6g; SODIUM 392mg; FIBER 7.9g; BETA-CAROTENE 6,686ug; VITAMIN C 51mg; CALCIUM 120mg; IRON 3.3mg; FOLATE 150ug; MAGNESIUM 80mg; ZINC 1.5mg; SELENIUM 4ug

Quick Corn and Bean Medley 🌿

SERVES 5

INGREDIENTS

2 cups fresh or frozen corn

1½ cups cooked great northern or cannellini beans* or 1 (15-ounce) can low-sodium or no-salt-added white beans, drained

1½ cups cooked kidney beans* or 1 (15-ounce) can low-sodium or no-salt-added kidney beans, drained

1 red bell pepper, diced

1 medium carrot, diced

1 large onion, diced

2 cloves garlic, chopped

1 medium potato, peeled and diced

3 cups water

No-salt seasoning blend, adjusted to taste, or 2 tablespoons Dr. Fuhrman's VegiZest

2 teaspoons dulse

1 teaspoon no-salt-added Mrs. Dash seasoning, or to taste

1 teaspoon herbes de Provence

14 ounces baby spinach

* Use ½ cup of each type of dried beans; see bean cooking instructions on page 19.

DIRECTIONS

Add all ingredients, except spinach, to a soup pot. Bring to a boil. Reduce heat, cover, and simmer for 20 minutes or until vegetables are tender. Add spinach and cook for an additional 5 minutes or until the spinach is wilted.

TO MAKE IN A CROCK POT:

Place all ingredients, except for spinach, in a crock pot and cook on low for 8 hours or high for 4 hours. Add the spinach to wilt 30 minutes before done.

PER SERVING: CALORIES 316; PROTEIN 19g; CARBOHYDRATES 63g; TOTAL FAT 1.8g; SATURATED FAT 0.3g; SODIUM 123mg; FIBER 15.1g; BETA-CAROTENE 8,014ug; VITAMIN C 81mg; CALCIUM 201mg; IRON 6.8mg; FOLATE 399ug; MAGNESIUM 170mg; ZINC 2.3mg; SELENIUM 5.5ug

Dulse is edible seaweed that is dried and powdered. It can be used as a condiment to lend some spice and salty flavor to soups and stews.

Cream of Asparagus Soup 🌿

INGREDIENTS

- 1 pound fresh asparagus, chopped
- No-salt seasoning blend, adjusted to taste, or 2 tablespoons Dr. Fuhrman's VegiZest
- 2 cups water
- 1 tablespoon Bragg Liquid Aminos
- 1 cup unsweetened soy, almond, or hemp milk
- ¼ cup raw cashews
- ¼ cup raw almonds
- 4 pitted dates
- Chopped fresh cilantro, for garnish

DIRECTIONS

Simmer asparagus, VegiZest or other no-salt seasoning blend, water, and Bragg Liquid Aminos in a soup pot until asparagus is tender.

Blend asparagus and liquid in a high-powered blender with soy milk, cashews, almonds, and dates, until smooth.

Garnish with cilantro before serving.

PER SERVING: CALORIES 223; PROTEIN 9g; CARBOHYDRATES 30g; TOTAL FAT 9.3g; SATURATED FAT 1.7g; CHOLESTEROL 0.1mg; SODIUM 225mg; FIBER 5.2g; BETA-CAROTENE 916ug; VITAMIN C 8mg; CALCIUM 80mg; IRON 4.2mg; FOLATE 86ug; MAGNESIUM 88mg; ZINC 1.8mg; SELENIUM 7.4ug

Creamy Zucchini Soup 🌿

SERVES 4

INGREDIENTS

....

1 large onion, chopped

3 cloves garlic, chopped

2 pounds zucchini (about 5 medium), chopped

1 teaspoon dried basil

½ teaspoon dried thyme

½ teaspoon dried oregano

4 cups no-salt-added or low-sodium vegetable broth

¼ cup raw cashews or ⅛ cup raw cashew butter

2 cups corn kernels (see Note)

4 cups baby spinach

¼ teaspoon black pepper, or to taste

DIRECTIONS

....

Add onion, garlic, zucchini, basil, thyme, oregano, and vegetable broth to a large soup pot. Bring to a boil, reduce heat, and simmer for 25 minutes or until zucchini is tender.

Pour into a food processor or high-powered blender (in batches, if necessary), add the cashews, and blend until smooth and creamy.

Return soup to the pot, add corn and baby spinach, bring to a simmer, and cook until spinach is wilted. Add water if needed to adjust consistency. Season with black pepper

NOTE: Use fresh or defrosted frozen corn kernels. If using fresh corn, boil 2 ears of corn until tender, about 4 minutes. Cut kernels from cobs with a sharp knife.

....

PER SERVING: CALORIES 195; PROTEIN 10g; CARBOHYDRATES 33g; TOTAL FAT 5.4g; SATURATED FAT 1.1g; SODIUM 431mg; FIBER 6.9g; BETA-CAROTENE 1,981ug; VITAMIN C 72mg; CALCIUM 102mg; IRON 3.3mg; FOLATE 165ug; MAGNESIUM 105mg; ZINC 1.8mg; SELENIUM 2.7ug

Dr. Fuhrman's Famous Anticancer Soup 🌿

SERVES 10

INGREDIENTS

....

1 cup dried split peas and beans

4 cups water

6–10 medium zucchini

5 pounds carrots, juiced (5–6 cups juice; see Note)

2 bunches celery, juiced (2 cups juice; see Note)

2 tablespoons Dr. Fuhrman's VegiZest

1 teaspoon Mrs. Dash no-salt seasoning

4 medium onions, chopped

3 leek stalks, coarsely chopped

2 bunches kale, collard greens, or other greens, tough stems and center ribs removed

1 cup raw cashews

2½ cups fresh mushrooms (shiitake, cremini, and/or white), chopped

DIRECTIONS

....

Place the split peas, beans, and water in a very large pot over low heat. Bring to a boil, reduce heat, and simmer. Add the zucchini whole to the pot. Add the carrot juice, celery juice, VegiZest, and Mrs. Dash.

Put the onions, leeks, and kale in a blender and blend with a little bit of the soup liquid. Pour this mixture into the soup pot.

Remove the softened zucchini with tongs and blend them in the blender with the cashews until creamy. Pour this mixture back into the soup pot. Add the mushrooms and continue to simmer the beans until soft, about 2 hours total cooking time.

NOTE: Use freshly juiced organic carrots and celery to maximize the flavor of this soup.

....

PER SERVING: CALORIES 322; PROTEIN 16g; CARBOHYDRATES 56g; TOTAL FAT 7.4g; SATURATED FAT 1.3g; SODIUM 130mg; FIBER 12g; BETA-CAROTENE 24,498ug; VITAMIN C 165mg; CALCIUM 236mg; IRON 5.6mg; FOLATE 174ug; MAGNESIUM 162mg; ZINC 2.8mg; SELENIUM 7.8ug

Ukrainian Sweet and Sour Cabbage Soup ✐

SERVES 4

INGREDIENTS

4–6 unsulfured prunes, pitted (reduce to 3 prunes for diabetic or weight-loss diets)

2 Granny Smith apples, cored and quartered

5 cups water, divided

1 large onion, chopped

1 cup chopped carrots

2 cups unsweetened soy, hemp, or almond milk

¼ cup dried split peas

¼ cup hulled barley

½ head cabbage, coarsely chopped

1 teaspoon dried basil

1 teaspoon dried oregano

½ teaspoon dried thyme

Black pepper to taste

3 tablespoons lemon juice

½ cup raw walnuts, toasted then finely chopped

1 teaspoon caraway seeds

DIRECTIONS

Blend the prunes, apples, and 2 cups of the water in a high-powered blender until smooth and creamy.

Add to a large soup pot along with the remaining water, onion, carrots, nondairy milk, split peas, barley, cabbage, basil, oregano, thyme, and black pepper. Bring to a boil, reduce heat, cover, and simmer for 1 hour.

Stir in lemon juice, chopped walnuts, and caraway seeds.

PER SERVING: CALORIES 363; PROTEIN 18g; CARBOHYDRATES 55g; TOTAL FAT 12.8g; SATURATED FAT 1.4g; SODIUM 122mg; FIBER 14.7g; BETA-CAROTENE 3,125ug; VITAMIN C 55mg; CALCIUM 164mg; IRON 4mg; FOLATE 134mg; MAGNESIUM 117mg; ZINC 2.1mg; SELENIUM 11.7ug

French Minted Pea Soup 🌿

SERVES 3

INGREDIENTS

- 10 ounces frozen green peas
- 1 small onion, chopped
- 1 clove garlic, chopped
- 1 bunch fresh mint leaves (save a few leaves for garnish)
- No-salt seasoning blend, adjusted to taste, or 3 tablespoons Dr. Fuhrman's VegiZest
- 3 cups water
- 3 dates, pitted
- ½ cup raw cashews or ¼ cup raw cashew butter
- ½ tablespoon Spike no-salt seasoning, or other no-salt seasoning to taste
- 4 teaspoons fresh lemon juice
- 4 cups shredded romaine lettuce or chopped baby spinach
- 2 tablespoons fresh snipped chives

DIRECTIONS

Simmer peas, onions, garlic, mint, and VegiZest or other no-salt seasoning blend in water for about 7 minutes.

Pour pea mixture into a high-powered blender or food processor. Add dates, cashews, no-salt seasoning, and lemon juice. Blend until smooth and creamy.

Add lettuce or spinach and let it wilt in hot liquid.

Pour into bowls and garnish with chives and mint leaves.

PER SERVING: CALORIES 301; PROTEIN 14g; CARBOHYDRATES 44g; TOTAL FAT 10.4g; SATURATED FAT 1.8g; SODIUM 180mg; FIBER 10.1g; BETA-CAROTENE 5,661ug; VITAMIN C 54mg; CALCIUM 150mg; IRON 8.4mg; FOLATE 219ug; MAGNESIUM 134mg; ZINC 2.7mg; SELENIUM 7.2ug

Golden Austrian Cauliflower Cream Soup

SERVES 4

INGREDIENTS

1 head cauliflower, cut into pieces

3 carrots, coarsely chopped

1 cup coarsely chopped celery

2 leeks, coarsely chopped

2 cloves garlic, minced

No-salt seasoning blend, adjusted to taste, or 2 tablespoons Dr. Fuhrman's VegiZest

2 cups carrot juice (2 pounds carrots, juiced)

4 cups water

½ teaspoon nutmeg

1 cup raw cashews or ½ cup raw cashew butter

5 cups chopped kale leaves or baby spinach

DIRECTIONS

Place all the ingredients, except the cashews and kale, in a pot. Cover and simmer for 15 minutes or until the vegetables are just tender. Steam the kale until tender. If you are using spinach, there is no need to steam it; it will wilt in the hot soup.

In a food processor or high-powered blender, blend two-thirds of the soup liquid and vegetables with the cashews until smooth and creamy. Return to the pot and stir in the steamed kale (or raw spinach).

PER SERVING: CALORIES 354; PROTEIN 13g; CARBOHYDRATES 46g; TOTAL FAT 16.7g; SATURATED FAT 3.4g; SODIUM 202mg; FIBER 9.1g; BETA-CAROTENE 18,003ug; VITAMIN C 102mg; CALCIUM 176mg; IRON 5.8mg; FOLATE 233ug; MAGNESIUM 182mg; ZINC 3mg; SELENIUM 6.8ug

Juicing Tip:
One pound of carrots will give you about 8 ounces of carrot juice.
Use organic carrots for the best flavor.

Cruciferous Vegetable Stew 🌿

INGREDIENTS

- 4 cups water
- 2½ cups carrot juice (2½ pounds carrots, juiced)
- ½ cup dried split peas
- ½ cup dried lentils
- ½ cup adzuki beans, soaked overnight
- 1 bunch kale, tough stems and center ribs removed and leaves coarsely chopped
- 1 bunch collard greens, tough stems and center ribs removed and leaves coarsely chopped
- 1 head broccoli, cut into florets
- 8 ounces shiitake mushrooms, cut in half
- 3 celery stalks, cut into 1-inch pieces
- 3 leeks, coarsely chopped
- 3 carrots, cut into 1-inch pieces
- 3 parsnips, cut into 1-inch pieces
- 3 medium onions, chopped
- 4 medium zucchini, cubed
- 4 cloves garlic, chopped
- 1 (28-ounce) can no-salt-added chopped tomatoes
- No-salt seasoning blend, adjusted to taste, or ¼ cup Dr. Fuhrman's VegiZest
- 2 tablespoons Mrs. Dash seasoning
- ¼ cup chopped fresh parsley
- 1 cup broccoli sprouts

DIRECTIONS

Place all the ingredients except the parsley and sprouts in a very large soup pot. Cover and bring to a simmer, cooking until the adzuki beans are tender, about 90 minutes.

In a food processor or high-powered blender, blend one-quarter of the soup until smooth. Return to the soup pot and stir in the parsley and broccoli sprouts.

PER SERVING: CALORIES 313; PROTEIN 18g; CARBOHYDRATES 64g; TOTAL FAT 1.4g; SATURATED FAT 0.2g; SODIUM 263mg; FIBER 15.6g; BETA-CAROTENE 26,932ug; VITAMIN C 114mg; CALCIUM 202mg; IRON 5mg; FOLATE 294ug; MAGNESIUM 105mg; ZINC 2.4mg; SELENIUM 6.6ug

Cruciferous vegetables are not only the most powerful anticancer foods in existence; they are also the most micronutrient-dense of all vegetables. Try to eat two servings of cruciferous vegetables daily.

The Cruciferous Vegetables Are:

Arugula	Cauliflower	Radishes
Bok choy	Collard greens	Red cabbage
Broccoli	Horseradish	Rutabaga leaf
Broccoli rabe	Kale	Swiss chard
Brussels sprouts	Kohlrabi	Turnip greens
Cabbage	Mustard greens	Watercress

Very Veggie Stew 🌿

>> Talia Fuhrman

The first time I made this stew, it was gone in a day. My whole family devoured it! It's super healthy, with interesting subtle flavors.

SERVES 6

INGREDIENTS

5 plum tomatoes, quartered

3 teaspoons olive oil, divided

3 cloves garlic, minced

1 large white onion, chopped

1 teaspoon cinnamon

1 teaspoon coriander

1 zucchini, chopped

1 yellow summer squash, chopped

1 red bell pepper, chopped

3 carrots, peeled and chopped

1 cup shiitake mushrooms

1½ cups cooked kidney or other beans* or 1 (15-ounce) can low-sodium or no-salt-added beans, drained

2 tablespoons fresh parsley, minced

1 tablespoon lemon juice

½ teaspoon garlic powder

½ teaspoon onion powder

No-salt seasoning blend, adjusted to taste, or 1 tablespoon Dr. Fuhrman's MatoZest

½ teaspoon Mrs. Dash or black pepper to taste

¼ cup toasted raw almonds, chopped (see box on next page)

* Use ½ cup dried beans; see bean cooking instructions on page 19.

DIRECTIONS

Preheat the oven to 475°F.

Place tomatoes on a nonstick baking pan and toss with 1 teaspoon olive oil. Bake for 20 minutes, until tomatoes are soft and beginning to brown. Remove from oven, cool, and chop coarsely. Set aside.

In a large pot over low heat, add garlic, onion, 2 teaspoons olive oil, and 1 tablespoon water. Cook until onions are translucent, about 5 to 8 minutes. Stir in cinnamon and coriander and heat for another few minutes. Add zucchini, yellow squash, red pepper, parsley, carrots, and mushrooms and cook for 8 to 10 minutes. Add water as needed. Stir in roasted tomatoes and beans and continue to cook over medium heat for 20 minutes, checking and stirring often. Add water and adjust heat as needed. Add lemon juice, garlic powder, onion powder, MatoZest or other no-salt seasoning blend, and black pepper. (Add seasonings gradually and adjust spice levels to your liking.) Cook for another few minutes and remove from heat. Let sit for 30 minutes. Stir in chopped almonds before serving.

PER SERVING: CALORIES 146; PROTEIN 11g; CARBOHYDRATES 25g; TOTAL FAT 3.1g; SATURATED FAT 0.4g; SODIUM 42mg; FIBER 7.1g; BETA-CAROTENE 3,769ug; VITAMIN C 59mg; CALCIUM 63mg; IRON 2.2mg; FOLATE 116ug; MAGNESIUM 53mg; ZINC 1.1mg; SELENIUM 2.5ug

Giving raw nuts and seeds a light toast in the oven enhances flavor and does not destroy food value or nutrients. Bake whole nuts in a 250°F oven for about 20 minutes, stirring occasionally until they are very lightly browned.

Persian Chickpea Stew 🌿

SERVES 4

INGREDIENTS

1 large eggplant, chopped into ¾-inch pieces

2 medium red bell peppers, coarsely chopped

1 large onion, chopped

4 medium zucchini, chopped into ¾-inch pieces

1 cup no-salt-added or low-sodium pasta sauce

2–4 cloves garlic, chopped

½ teaspoon cinnamon

½ teaspoon ground coriander

½ teaspoon turmeric

1 cup carrot juice (1 pound carrots, juiced)

½ cup water

1½ cups cooked garbanzo beans* (chickpeas) or 1 (15-ounce) can no-salt-added or low-sodium garbanzo beans, drained

⅓ cup fresh parsley, chopped

12 ounces fresh spinach

* Use ½ cup dried beans; see cooking instructions on page 19.

DIRECTIONS

Sauté eggplant, peppers, and onion in a small amount of water, covered, for 5 minutes, stirring occasionally. Add zucchini, cover, and cook an additional 3 minutes. Add the pasta sauce, garlic, cinnamon, coriander, turmeric, carrot juice, water, and garbanzo beans. Cover and cook over low heat 25 minutes, or until eggplant is tender.

Add half the parsley and simmer 30 seconds. Taste and adjust seasonings. Stir in remaining parsley and spinach. Spinach will wilt in hot stew.

NOTE: May be served hot or at room temperature.

PER SERVING: CALORIES 312; PROTEIN 15g; CARBOHYDRATES 58g; TOTAL FAT 5.9g; SATURATED FAT 0.8g; SODIUM 147mg; FIBER 15.8g; BETA-CAROTENE 12,282ug; VITAMIN C 159mg; CALCIUM 210mg; IRON 6.6mg; FOLATE 409ug; MAGNESIUM 186mg; ZINC 2.7mg; SELENIUM 5.4ug

Shiitake Portobello Stew 🌱

SERVES 4

INGREDIENTS

1 large onion, diced into ½-inch pieces

1 red bell pepper, seeded and thinly sliced

2 teaspoons chopped fresh rosemary

No-salt seasoning blend, adjusted to taste, or 2 tablespoons Dr. Fuhrman's MatoZest

⅛ teaspoon crushed red pepper flakes

1 pound portobello mushrooms, sliced ⅜ inch thick

1 pound shiitake mushrooms, sliced

2 cloves garlic, minced

3 tablespoons tomato paste

4 cups low-sodium or no-salt-added mushroom or vegetable broth

1 tablespoon sherry vinegar

2 tablespoons fresh parsley or tarragon, chopped

DIRECTIONS

Water-sauté the onion, bell pepper, and rosemary, stirring occasionally until tender, about 8 minutes. Season with MatoZest or other no-salt seasoning blend and red pepper flakes.

Add the mushrooms and sauté until tender and juicy, about 5 minutes. Add the garlic, tomato paste, vegetable broth, and sherry vinegar. Simmer over low heat for 15 minutes. Garnish with parsley or tarragon.

PER SERVING: CALORIES 124; PROTEIN 9g; CARBOHYDRATES 17g; TOTAL FAT 1.7g; SATURATED FAT 0.1g; SODIUM 139mg; FIBER 4g; BETA-CAROTENE 1,289ug; VITAMIN C 53mg; CALCIUM 35mg; IRON 2.2mg; FOLATE 60ug; MAGNESIUM 36mg; ZINC 1.4mg; SELENIUM 22.2ug

Shiitake Watercress Soup 🌿

INGREDIENTS

2 large leeks, white and pale green parts only, washed thoroughly and cut into ½-inch slices

3 medium carrots, peeled and chopped

3 cloves garlic, chopped

3 cups shiitake mushrooms, sliced

6 cups low-sodium or no-salt-added vegetable broth

3 cups cooked white beans* or 2 (15-ounce) cans low-sodium or no-salt-added white beans, drained

5 cups watercress, stems removed

1 teaspoon herbes de Provence

Black pepper to taste

* Use 1 cup dried beans; see bean cooking instructions on page 19.

DIRECTIONS

Heat ⅛ cup water in a soup pot. Add leeks, carrot, and garlic and water-sauté until tender, about 3 minutes. Add mushrooms and cook an additional 3 minutes or until mushroom juices are released. Add vegetable broth, beans, watercress, and herbes de Provence and simmer for 15 minutes.

Ladle half of the soup into a food processor or high-powered blender and puree until smooth. Return to pot. Season with pepper.

NOTE: *For a nonvegan option, add 4 ounces of chicken along with the vegetable broth, simmer until cooked through, remove from pot, slice or shred into small pieces, and return to soup.*

PER SERVING: CALORIES 284; PROTEIN 23g; CARBOHYDRATES 47g; TOTAL FAT 3.3g; SATURATED FAT 0.9g; SODIUM 173mg; FIBER 12.4g; BETA-CAROTENE 5,434ug; VITAMIN C 30mg; CALCIUM 204mg; IRON 5.1mg; FOLATE 188ug; MAGNESIUM 104mg; ZINC 2.1mg; SELENIUM 13.3ug

Tomato Bisque

SERVES 4

INGREDIENTS

- 3 cups carrot juice (3 pounds carrots, juiced)
- 1½ pounds fresh tomatoes, chopped or 1 (26-ounce) BPA-free carton no-salt-added chopped tomatoes
- ¼ cup unsalted, unsulfured dried tomatoes, chopped
- 2 celery stalks, chopped
- 1 small onion, chopped
- 1 leek, chopped
- 1 large shallot, chopped
- 3 cloves garlic, chopped
- No-salt seasoning blend, adjusted to taste, or 2 tablespoons Dr. Fuhrman's MatoZest
- 1 teaspoon dried thyme, crumbled
- 1 small bay leaf
- ½ cup raw almonds
- ¼ cup hemp seeds
- ¼ cup chopped fresh basil
- 5 ounces baby spinach

DIRECTIONS

In a large saucepan, add all ingredients except the almonds, hemp seeds, basil, and spinach. Simmer for 30 minutes. Discard the bay leaf.

Remove 2 cups of the vegetables with a slotted spoon and set aside. Puree the remaining soup with the almonds and hemp seeds in a high-powered blender until smooth. Return the pureed soup along with the reserved vegetables to the pot. Stir in the basil and spinach and heat until spinach is wilted.

PER SERVING: CALORIES 300; PROTEIN 16g; CARBOHYDRATES 43g; TOTAL FAT 12g; SATURATED FAT 1g; SODIUM 208mg; FIBER 10g; BETA-CAROTENE 20,201ug; VITAMIN C 58mg; CALCIUM 211mg; IRON 4.9mg; FOLATE 147ug; MAGNESIUM 148mg; ZINC 1.8mg; SELENIUM 3ug

To store fresh basil, place stems in a glass with 1 inch of water and store at room temperature. If you change the water daily, the basil will stay fresh for several days.

Three Sisters Harvest Stew 🌿

SERVES 4

INGREDIENTS

1 medium onion, chopped

2 cloves garlic, chopped

1 jalapeño chili, seeded and minced

1½ cups cooked kidney or pinto beans* or 1 (15-ounce) can low-sodium or no-salt-added kidney beans, drained

½ cup green bell pepper, cut into strips

½ cup red bell pepper, cut into strips

2 cups corn kernels

2 cups low-sodium or no-salt-added vegetable stock

3 cups chopped acorn, butternut, or carnival squash, peeled and cut into ¾-inch chunks

1 teaspoon ground cumin

1½ cups diced tomatoes, fresh or packaged in BPA-free cartons

1 teaspoon dried oregano

⅛ teaspoon ground pepper

5 ounces spinach

¼ cup raw pumpkin seeds, lightly toasted

* Use ½ cup dried beans; see bean cooking instructions on page 19.

DIRECTIONS

Heat 2 tablespoons water in a soup pot, add the onion, and sauté until tender. Add the garlic and jalapeño and continue to sauté for an additional minute.

Add remaining ingredients except spinach and pumpkin seeds. Bring to a boil, reduce heat, and simmer until all the vegetables are tender, about 25 minutes. Add additional vegetable broth if needed to adjust consistency. Stir in spinach and heat until wilted.

Serve topped with toasted pumpkin seeds.

PER SERVING: CALORIES 378; PROTEIN 22g; CARBOHYDRATES 66g; TOTAL FAT 8g; SATURATED FAT 1.7g; CHOLESTEROL 8.4mg; SODIUM 86mg; FIBER 11.8g; BETA-CAROTENE 4,406ug; VITAMIN C 108mg; CALCIUM 141mg; IRON 6.1mg; FOLATE 258ug; MAGNESIUM 173mg; ZINC 3.3mg; SELENIUM 9.2ug

In Native American mythology, squash, corn, and beans are known as the "three sisters." Interplanting corn, beans, and squash in the same mounds enhances their growth and was widespread among American Indian farming societies. Corn acts as a trellis for climbing beans, which nourish the soil with nitrogen, and squash vines shade the shallow corn and bean roots.

Too-Busy-To-Cook Vegetable Bean Soup

SERVES 6

INGREDIENTS

3 cups frozen corn, thawed, divided

2 cups unsweetened soy, hemp, or almond milk

4 cups frozen chopped kale

2 cups frozen chopped broccoli

2 cups frozen oriental vegetables

2 cups carrot juice

3 cups cooked beans* or 2 (15-ounce) cans low-sodium or no-salt-added beans

No-salt seasoning blend, adjusted to taste, or 2 tablespoons Dr. Fuhrman's VegiZest

* Use 1 cup dried beans; see bean cooking instructions on page 19.

DIRECTIONS

Blend 1½ cups of the corn with the milk. Pour into a large pot. Add remaining ingredients and bring to a boil. Reduce heat, cover, and simmer for 35 minutes.

To make an extra creamy version of this recipe, blend half of the cooked soup until creamy and add back to the pot.

PER SERVING: CALORIES 323; PROTEIN 19g; CARBOHYDRATES 61g; TOTAL FAT 3.4g; SATURATED FAT 0.5g; SODIUM 126mg; FIBER 15.5g; BETA-CAROTENE 8,373ug; VITAMIN C 66mg; CALCIUM 181mg; IRON 4.9mg; FOLATE 230ug; MAGNESIUM 135mg; ZINC 2.3mg; SELENIUM 8ug

> The longest lived societies in the world eat beans almost every day.

West African Lentil Okra Stew

SERVES 8

INGREDIENTS

2 cups red lentils

2 tablespoons tomato paste (see box)

½ cup smooth, natural, no-salt peanut butter, at room temperature

No-salt seasoning blend, adjusted to taste, or ¼ cup Dr. Fuhrman's MatoZest

4 cups carrot juice (4 pounds carrots, juiced)

2 cups frozen chopped onion

16 ounces frozen okra, thawed and cut in half crosswise

16 ounces frozen chopped kale or collard greens

1½ cups chopped tomatoes, fresh or packaged in BPA-free cartons

1 medium sweet potato, chopped

4 cloves garlic, minced or pressed

1 tablespoon chili powder

Pinch of cayenne pepper

DIRECTIONS

In a large saucepan, simmer red lentils in 3 cups of water for 15 minutes.

In a mixing bowl, whisk together tomato paste, peanut butter, MatoZest or other no-salt seasoning blend, and carrot juice, then add to simmering lentils.

Add remaining ingredients and bring to a boil. Reduce heat, cover, and simmer for about 20 minutes. Uncover and simmer another 20 minutes.

PER SERVING: CALORIES 399; PROTEIN 23g; CARBOHYDRATES 62g; TOTAL FAT 9.5g; SATURATED FAT 1.9g; SODIUM 125mg; FIBER 21g; BETA-CAROTENE 18,428ug; VITAMIN C 45mg; CALCIUM 211mg; IRON 6.2mg; FOLATE 354ug; MAGNESIUM 150mg; ZINC 3.6mg; SELENIUM 7.2ug

I recommend that people avoid canned tomato products because tomatoes are acidic, which can cause a significant amount of BPA (Bisphenol A) to leach into the food from the lining of the can. Look for tomato paste packaged in glass jars. The Bionaturæ company makes this type of product.

Tuscan Cannellini Bean Soup with a Chiffonade of Collard Greens 🌿

INGREDIENTS

- 1 cup unsulfured, unsalted dried tomatoes
- ½ cup unsweetened soy, hemp, or almond milk
- 1 cup finely chopped onions
- 2 cloves garlic, minced
- 1 tablespoon fresh oregano
- 1 tablespoon fresh rosemary
- 1½ cups cooked cannellini beans* or 1 (15-ounce) can no-salt-added or low-sodium cannellini beans
- 1½ cups diced tomatoes, fresh or packaged in BPA-free cartons
- 1½ cups no-salt-added tomato puree
- 3 cups no-salt-added or low-sodium vegetable broth
- 1 cup water
- No-salt seasoning blend, adjusted to taste, or 1 tablespoon Dr. Fuhrman's MatoZest
- 6 cups collard greens, cut chiffonade (very thinly sliced)
- 2 tablespoons sherry vinegar or Dr. Fuhrman's Black Fig Vinegar
- ½ teaspoon freshly ground black pepper
- 2 tablespoons fresh basil

* Use ½ cup dried beans; see bean cooking instructions on page 19.

DIRECTIONS

Soak the dried tomatoes in soy milk for 1 hour to soften. Drain, reserving soy milk. Chop tomatoes finely and set aside.

Water-sauté onions and garlic in a large pot, stirring constantly. Add dried tomatoes, reserved soy milk, oregano, rosemary, beans, diced tomatoes, tomato puree, broth, water, and MatoZest or other no-salt seasoning blend. Bring to a boil. Lower heat and simmer for about 20 minutes. Add the sliced greens just before serving and bring to a simmer, no longer than 2 minutes.

Before serving, stir in vinegar, black pepper, and fresh basil.

PER SERVING: CALORIES 247; PROTEIN 17g; CARBOHYDRATES 43g; TOTAL FAT 3.7g; SATURATED FAT 1g; CHOLESTEROL 8.4mg; SODIUM 282mg; FIBER 8.5g; BETA-CAROTENE 3,565ug; VITAMIN C 35mg; CALCIUM 161mg; IRON 5.2mg; FOLATE 148ug; MAGNESIUM 85mg; ZINC 2.4mg; SELENIUM 9.4ug

Chiffonade is a term for slicing herbs and leafy vegetables into long, thin strips. Stack and roll a small pile of leaves and then slice them into thin ribbons. Adding a chiffonade of Swiss chard, collard greens, mustard greens, kale, or watercress during the last few minutes of cooking is a nice finishing touch for soups and hot vegetable dishes.

Yellow Lentil Dal with Mango 🌿

SERVES 4

INGREDIENTS

- 1 cup dry yellow lentils, rinsed
- 4 cups water
- ½ teaspoon ground turmeric
- 1 medium onion, chopped
- 4 cloves garlic, minced
- 1 tablespoon minced fresh ginger
- ½ teaspoon ground coriander
- 1 teaspoon ground cumin
- ¼ teaspoon black pepper
- 2 mangoes, peeled and diced
- 3 cups coarsely chopped spinach
- ½ cup chopped fresh cilantro

DIRECTIONS

Combine lentils, water, and turmeric in a large saucepan. Bring to a boil, reduce heat, partially cover, and cook, stirring occasionally, for 15 minutes.

Meanwhile, water-sauté onion until almost tender, about 3 minutes. Add garlic and ginger and cook for an additional 2 minutes. Add coriander, cumin, and black pepper.

Stir the onion mixture and mangoes into the lentils. Return to a simmer and cook, stirring occasionally, until lentils are very tender, about 15 minutes. Stir in spinach and cilantro and heat until spinach is wilted.

PER SERVING: CALORIES 265; PROTEIN 14g; CARBOHYDRATES 52g; TOTAL FAT 1.1g; SATURATED FAT 0.2g; SODIUM 38mg; FIBER 18.1g; BETA-CAROTENE 2,070ug; VITAMIN C 44mg; CALCIUM 91mg; IRON 4.8mg; FOLATE 300ug; MAGNESIUM 95mg; ZINC 2.6mg; SELENIUM 5.5ug

Gazpacho Summer Soup 🍃

SERVES 3

INGREDIENTS

- 1 large cucumber, peeled and sliced into large pieces
- 1 large red bell pepper, seeded and sliced into large pieces
- 1½ cups diced fresh tomatoes, fresh or packaged in BPA-free cartons
- 1 cup low-sodium roasted red peppers, in vinegar, drained
- 2 cups no-salt-added or low-sodium tomato juice
- 1½ cups mild or medium no-salt-added or low-sodium salsa
- ½ cup fresh cilantro
- 2 tablespoons red wine vinegar
- No-salt seasoning blend, adjusted to taste, or 1 tablespoon Dr. Fuhrman's MatoZest
- Additional cucumber slices

DIRECTIONS

Place cucumbers and fresh red bell peppers in a food processor. Pulse until chopped in small pieces. Add tomatoes and roasted red peppers. Pulse again until finely chopped. Add tomato juice, salsa, cilantro, vinegar, and MatoZest or other no-salt seasoning blend and pulse until well mixed.

Cover and chill for at least 2 hours to allow flavors to mingle.

Before serving, garnish with cucumber slices. Serve chilled.

PER SERVING: CALORIES 106; PROTEIN 10g; CARBOHYDRATES 23g; TOTAL FAT 0.9g; SATURATED FAT 0.1g; SODIUM 51mg; FIBER 5.7g; BETA-CAROTENE 3,566ug; VITAMIN C 176mg; CALCIUM 63mg; IRON 2.2mg; FOLATE 121ug; MAGNESIUM 63mg; ZINC 0.9mg; SELENIUM 0.8ug

Watermelon Gazpacho 🌿

SERVES 6

INGREDIENTS

- 1 seedless watermelon, ½ cubed and ½ diced
- 5 cucumbers, 3 chopped, 2 diced
- 1 red bell pepper, finely diced
- ¼ cup minced shallots
- 3 organic limes, juiced and zested
- ½ bunch mint, finely chopped

DIRECTIONS

Puree cubed watermelon and chopped cucumbers in a blender. You will need to work in batches. Allow to chill at least 1 hour. Add diced watermelon and cucumber to the juice along with red pepper, shallots, lime juice, zest, and mint.

PER SERVING: CALORIES 277; PROTEIN 7g; CARBOHYDRATES 70g; TOTAL FAT 1.5g; SATURATED FAT 0.2g; SODIUM 15mg; FIBER 5.7g; BETA-CAROTENE 2,567ug; VITAMIN C 79mg; CALCIUM 119mg; IRON 3.6mg; FOLATE 51ug; MAGNESIUM 115mg; ZINC 1.4mg; SELENIUM 3.9ug

Black Bean and Butternut Squash Chili 🌿

SERVES 5

INGREDIENTS

2 cups chopped onions

3 cloves garlic, chopped

2½ cups chopped (½-inch pieces) butternut squash

4½ cups cooked black beans* or 3 (15-ounce) cans low-sodium or no-salt-added black beans, drained

2 tablespoons chili powder

2 teaspoons ground cumin

2½ cups low-sodium or no-salt-added vegetable broth

1½ cups diced tomatoes, fresh or packaged in BPA-free cartons

1 bunch Swiss chard, tough stems removed, chopped

* Use 1½ cups dried beans; see bean cooking instructions on page 19.

DIRECTIONS

Add all ingredients, except Swiss chard, to a large pot. Bring to a boil, reduce heat, and simmer, uncovered, until squash is tender, about 20 minutes.

Stir in Swiss chard and simmer until chard is tender, about 4 minutes longer.

PER SERVING: CALORIES 379; PROTEIN 24g; CARBOHYDRATES 68g; TOTAL FAT 4.2g; SATURATED FAT 1.1g; CHOLESTEROL 8.4mg; SODIUM 177mg; FIBER 19g; BETA-CAROTENE 6,685ug; VITAMIN C 44mg; CALCIUM 151mg; IRON 6mg; FOLATE 300ug; MAGNESIUM 190mg; ZINC 3.4mg; SELENIUM 9.5ug

Crock Pot Mushroom Chili 🍃

SERVES 4

INGREDIENTS

1 onion, diced

2 cloves garlic, minced

1 green bell pepper, chopped

1 cup fresh or frozen corn kernels

1 zucchini, diced

8 ounces mushrooms, sliced

3 cups diced tomatoes, fresh or packaged in BPA-free cartons

3 cups cooked kidney or pinto beans* or 2 (15-ounce) cans low-sodium or no-salt-added kidney beans

½ cup water

2 tablespoons chili powder

2 teaspoons cumin

½ teaspoon oregano

Dash of cayenne pepper, or to taste

* Use 1 cup dried beans; see cooking instructions on page 19.

DIRECTIONS

Combine all ingredients in a crock pot. Cover and cook on low for 7 hours.

PER SERVING: CALORIES 286; PROTEIN 21g; CARBOHYDRATES 55g; TOTAL FAT 2.5g; SATURATED FAT 0.4g; SODIUM 62mg; FIBER 14.9g; BETA-CAROTENE 1,334ug; VITAMIN C 60mg; CALCIUM 105mg; IRON 4.7mg; FOLATE 243ug; MAGNESIUM 105mg; ZINC 2.4mg; SELENIUM 7.7ug

Goji Chili Stew 🌿

INGREDIENTS

3 cups diced tomatoes, fresh or packaged in BPA-free cartons

5 cups chopped fresh broccoli or 1 pound frozen chopped broccoli

1 cup fresh or frozen chopped onions

2½ cups corn kernels

½ cup goji berries

2 large zucchini, diced

4 ounces chopped mild green chilies

4 teaspoons chili powder, or more to taste

2 teaspoons cumin

3 cloves garlic, minced

1½ cups cooked pinto beans* or 1 (15-ounce) can low-sodium or no-salt-added pinto beans, drained

1½ cups cooked black beans* or 1 (15-ounce) can low-sodium or no-salt-added black beans, drained

1½ cup cooked red kidney beans* or 1 (15-ounce) can low-sodium or no-salt-added kidney beans, drained

*Use ½ cup of each type of dried beans; see bean cooking instructions on page 19.

DIRECTIONS

Cover and simmer all ingredients, except beans, for 20 minutes. Add beans and cook for an additional 10 minutes.

NOTE: The Spiced Sweet Potato Cornbread (page 266) makes a nice side dish.

PER SERVING: CALORIES 495; PROTEIN 32g; CARBOHYDRATES 95g; TOTAL FAT 2.9g; SATURATED FAT 0.5g; SODIUM 170mg; FIBER 26.4g; BETA-CAROTENE 1,244ug; VITAMIN C 113mg; CALCIUM 181mg; IRON 8.9mg; FOLATE 477ug; MAGNESIUM 178mg; ZINC 3.6mg; SELENIUM 8.2ug

MAIN DISHES

Recipes recommended for aggressive weight-loss and diabetic diets and for people with metabolic syndrome are marked with 🌿.

MAIN DISHES

To really experience all the pleasures and benefits that a nutritarian diet has to offer, you must learn to make nutrient-rich meals in your own kitchen. The recipes included in this cookbook will help you understand and master the basic techniques and principles of high-nutrient food preparation, but you can switch around foods and adjust the recipes to reflect your own tastes and lifestyle.

Different ingredients and different spice and herb combinations can be used to healthfully reflect your cultural or personal food preferences. In the Italian culture, tomatoes, greens, beans, and peppers are mixed with garlic, onion, basil, oregano, and thyme. In Mexican cooking, corn, squash, jicama, avocado, beans, and hot peppers are mixed with cumin, chili powders, lime, cilantro, cinnamon, and garlic. Asian cuisines take broccoli, bok choy, cabbage, and mushrooms and mix them up with ginger, garlic, scallions, lemongrass, mint, Szechuan peppers, sesame seeds, and rice vinegar. If you enjoy Indian food, pair cauliflower, peas, tomato, and spinach with turmeric, cumin, curry blends, garam marsala, ginger, garlic, onion, and coriander.

ENHANCING FLAVORS

Many foods combine particularly well with certain herbs and spices and other seasonings.

ASPARAGUS
garlic, lemon juice, vinegar, chives, thyme

BEANS, DRIED
bay leaf, garlic, marjoram, onion, oregano, cumin, chili powder

BEANS, GREEN
lemon juice, marjoram, dill, nutmeg, black pepper, oregano

BEETS
lemon juice

BROCCOLI
lemon juice, garlic, dill, oregano, red pepper flakes

CABBAGE
fennel, caraway seeds, black pepper, Creole seasoning

CARROTS
parsley, mint, dill, ginger, cumin

CAULIFLOWER
paprika, curry powder, Italian seasonings, caraway seeds

CORN
black pepper, green bell pepper, fresh basil, fresh cilantro

CUCUMBERS
dill, chives, vinegar

GREENS
onion, garlic, hot pepper flakes, black pepper, lemon juice, vinegar

PEAS
mint, black pepper, parsley, onion

SQUASH AND SWEET POTATOES
onion, nutmeg, ginger, cinnamon, lemon juice

TOMATOES
basil, garlic, oregano, marjoram, onion

Thai Vegetable Curry 🌿

INGREDIENTS

4 cloves garlic, finely chopped

2 tablespoons finely chopped fresh ginger

2 tablespoons chopped fresh basil

2 tablespoons chopped fresh cilantro

2 cups carrot juice (2 pounds carrots, juiced)

1 red bell pepper, seeded and thinly sliced

1 large eggplant, peeled, if desired, and cut into 1-inch cubes

2 cups green beans, cut in 2-inch pieces

3 cups sliced shiitake mushrooms

1 (8-ounce) can bamboo shoots, drained

¼ teaspoon crushed red pepper flakes, or adjusted to taste

1 teaspoon curry powder

2 cups watercress leaves, divided

3 tablespoons unsalted, natural, chunky peanut butter

2 pounds firm tofu, cut into ¼-inch-thick slices

½ cup light coconut milk

Basil or cilantro leaves, for garnish

DIRECTIONS

Place the garlic, ginger, basil, cilantro, carrot juice, bell pepper, eggplant, green beans, mushrooms, bamboo shoots, crushed red pepper, curry powder, and 1 cup of the watercress in a wok or large skillet. Bring to a boil, cover, and simmer, stirring occasionally, until all the vegetables are tender. Mix in the peanut butter. Add the tofu, bring to a simmer, and toss until hot. Add the coconut milk and heat through. Top with the remaining 1 cup watercress. Garnish with basil or cilantro leaves, if desired.

May be served over brown rice or quinoa.

PER SERVING: CALORIES 375; PROTEIN 15g; CARBOHYDRATES 48g; TOTAL FAT 16.9g; SATURATED FAT 6.1g; SODIUM 108mg; FIBER 8.6g; BETA-CAROTENE 8,642ug; VITAMIN C 51mg; CALCIUM 205mg; IRON 5.3mg; FOLATE 114ug; MAGNESIUM 138mg; ZINC 3mg; SELENIUM 26.3ug

Asian Vegetable Stir-Fry 🌿

This recipe looks harder than it is. It is well worth the time it takes to prepare and is great for guests. Beans or small pieces of chicken breast or shrimp can also be stir-fried with the vegetables.

SERVES 4

INGREDIENTS

14 ounces extra-firm tofu, cubed

1 teaspoon Bragg Liquid Aminos or low-sodium soy sauce

¼ teaspoon crushed red pepper flakes

2 tablespoons Spike no-salt seasoning (or other no-salt seasoning blend, adjusted to taste)

½ cup brown rice or wild rice

¼ cup unhulled sesame seeds

FOR THE SAUCE:

¼ cup unsulfured, dried apricots, soaked overnight in ½ cup water to cover

¼ cup unsalted, natural peanut butter or raw cashew butter

2 tablespoons fresh chopped ginger

4 cloves garlic, chopped

No-salt seasoning blend, adjusted to taste, or 1 tablespoon Dr. Fuhrman's VegiZest

¼ cup Dr. Fuhrman's Black Fig Vinegar (see Note)

1 teaspoon arrowroot powder

¼ teaspoon crushed red pepper flakes

FOR THE VEGETABLES:

2 tablespoons water

1 medium onion, cut into wedges and separated into 1-inch strips

4 cups small broccoli florets

2 medium carrots, cut diagonally into ⅓-inch pieces

4 medium red bell peppers, seeded and cut into 1-inch squares

1 cup sugar snap peas or snow peas, strings removed

2 cups bok choy, cut in bite-size pieces

3 cups fresh mushrooms (shiitake, porcini and/or cremini), stems removed

1 pound fresh spinach

½ cup raw cashews, coarsely chopped

1¼ pounds romaine lettuce, shredded

DIRECTIONS

Marinate the tofu for 30 minutes in the liquid aminos, red pepper flakes, and Spike. While the tofu marinates, combine rice and 1¼ cups water in a saucepan. Bring to a boil. Reduce heat and cover. Simmer 30 minutes or until water is absorbed. Set aside.

Preheat the oven to 350°F. Toss the marinated tofu with the sesame seeds. Bake the sesame-coated tofu in a nonstick baking pan for 30 to 40 minutes, until golden.

To make the sauce, place the soaked apricots with the soaking liquid, peanut butter, ginger, garlic, VegiZest or other no-salt seasoning blend, vinegar, arrowroot powder, and red pepper flakes in a food processor or high-powered blender and blend until smooth. Transfer to a small bowl and set aside.

Heat water in a large pan and water-sauté the onion, broccoli, carrots, bell peppers, and peas for 5 minutes, adding more water as necessary to keep vegetables from scorching. Add the bok choy and mushrooms, cover, and simmer until the vegetables are just tender. Remove the cover and cook off most of the water. Add the spinach and toss until wilted.

Add the sauce and stir until all the vegetables are glazed and the sauce is hot and bubbly, about 1 minute. Mix in the cashews and baked tofu. Serve the stir-fry over the shredded lettuce along with ¼ cup rice per person.

NOTE: If you don't have Black Fig Vinegar, blend 4 unsulfured dried figs with ½ cup rice vinegar in a high-powered blender until smooth.

PER SERVING: CALORIES 386; PROTEIN 17g; CARBOHYDRATES 51g; TOTAL FAT 16.2g; SATURATED FAT 2.9g; SODIUM 190mg; FIBER 11g; BETA-CAROTENE 11,814ug; VITAMIN C 223mg; CALCIUM 319mg; IRON 7.9mg; FOLATE 433ug; MAGNESIUM 220mg; ZINC 3.6mg; SELENIUM 19.5ug

Mushrooms and Beans over Crispy Kale 🌿

SERVES 2

INGREDIENTS

FOR THE MUSHROOMS AND BEANS:

Small amount of olive oil

2–4 garlic cloves, chopped

1 shallot, chopped

1 pound mixed mushrooms (portobello, cremini, shiitake), sliced or quartered

1 cup cooked kidney beans* or canned no-salt-added or low-sodium
kidney beans, drained

½ cup low-sodium or no-salt-added vegetable broth

1 tablespoon sherry vinegar or balsamic vinegar

½ teaspoon fresh thyme, chopped

⅛ teaspoon black pepper

* Use ⅓ cup dried beans; see cooking instructions on page 19.

FOR THE SAUCE:

1¼ cups low-sodium or no-salt-added vegetable broth, divided

1 tablespoon tomato paste

¼ cup raisins (reduce to 2 tablespoons for diabetic and weight-loss diets)

2 teaspoons arrowroot powder

FOR THE CRISPY KALE:

Small amount of olive oil

1 bunch kale, tough stems and center ribs removed, chopped

DIRECTIONS

FOR THE MUSHROOMS AND BEANS:

Rub a large nonstick skillet with a small amount of olive oil and heat over medium-high heat. Add garlic, shallots, and mushrooms and cook, stirring frequently, until mushrooms are tender and liquid is evaporated.

Add kidney beans and vegetable broth and cook until heated through. Stir in vinegar, thyme, and black pepper. Cover and set aside.

FOR THE SAUCE:

Heat 1 cup of the vegetable broth in small saucepan. Add tomato paste and raisins and simmer on low heat for 3 minutes. Whisk arrowroot into remaining ¼ cup vegetable broth. Add to sauce and heat until mixture is slightly thickened.

FOR THE CRISPY KALE:

Preheat the oven to 350°F. Rub a baking dish with a small amount of olive oil. Spread kale leaves on the baking pan, making sure not to overlap the pieces. This will help the kale to crisp evenly. Bake for 20 minutes until the edges start to get crispy.

Serve mushrooms and kidney beans on a bed of crispy kale topped with sauce.

PER SERVING: CALORIES 301; PROTEIN 22g; CARBOHYDRATES 55g; TOTAL FAT 3.1g; SATURATED FAT 0.6g; SODIUM 150mg; FIBER 10.3g; BETA-CAROTENE 6,558ug; VITAMIN C 94mg; CALCIUM 162mg; IRON 5.4mg; FOLATE 186ug; MAGNESIUM 95mg; ZINC 2.7mg; SELENIUM 23.4ug

Pistachio-Crusted Tempeh with Balsamic-Glazed Shiitakes 🌿

INGREDIENTS

8 ounces tempeh, diagonally sliced as thinly as possible

1 pound shiitake mushrooms, stemmed and thinly sliced

FOR THE MARINADE:

2 cloves garlic, minced

1 tablespoon chopped fresh basil

1 tablespoon chopped fresh cilantro

Pinch of hot pepper flakes

1 cup low-sodium or no-salt-added vegetable broth

2 tablespoons balsamic vinegar

1 teaspoon Bragg Liquid Aminos or low-sodium soy sauce

FOR THE CRUST:

1 cup shelled pistachios

4 tablespoons cornmeal

2 tablespoons nutritional yeast

1 teaspoon onion powder

1 teaspoon garlic powder

DIRECTIONS

Place sliced tempeh in a saucepan with water to cover and simmer for 10 minutes.

Combine all ingredients for marinade. Remove tempeh from water and add to marinade. Marinate for at least 1 hour.

Preheat the oven to 375°F. Process pistachios in a food processor until finely chopped. Add remaining crust ingredients and pulse until thoroughly mixed. Place in a large shallow bowl. Remove tempeh from marinade and drain. Reserve marinade. Dip tempeh in crust mixture to coat.

Place crusted tempeh and sliced mushrooms side by side on a rimmed baking sheet. Spoon 2–3 tablespoons of marinade over mushrooms. Bake for 13 minutes or until mushrooms are soft, turning occasionally.

Simmer remaining marinade for 2 minutes. Drizzle tempeh and mushrooms with marinade before serving.

PER SERVING: CALORIES 374; PROTEIN 24g; CARBOHYDRATES 30g; TOTAL FAT 20.7g; SATURATED FAT 3.1g; SODIUM 98mg; FIBER 6.1g; BETA-CAROTENE 173ug; VITAMIN C 5mg; CALCIUM 120mg; IRON 4.7mg; FOLATE 225ug; MAGNESIUM 109mg; ZINC 2.4mg; SELENIUM 14.2ug

Spicy Thai Braised Kale and Tofu ✿

SERVES 4

INGREDIENTS

16 ounces extra-firm tofu, drained well, cut into 1-inch cubes

1 cup finely chopped onion

1 tablespoon grated fresh ginger

1 small jalapeño pepper, seeded and minced

1 teaspoon chili powder

2 cups no-salt-added or low-sodium vegetable broth

½ cup unsalted, natural peanut butter

2 tablespoons tomato paste

No-salt seasoning blend, adjusted to taste, or 2 tablespoons Dr. Fuhrman's MatoZest

1 bunch kale, tough stems and center ribs removed and leaves chopped

1 tablespoon fresh lime juice

4 scallions, thinly sliced

DIRECTIONS

Preheat the oven to 350°F. Place tofu cubes on a lightly oiled baking dish and bake for 30 minutes, turning after 15 minutes.

Heat a large sauté pan and add onion, ginger, and jalapeño pepper. Cook until onion has softened, adding 1–2 teaspoons of water as needed to prevent sticking. Add chili powder and cook 1 more minute.

Whisk in vegetable broth, peanut butter, tomato paste, and MatoZest or other no-salt seasoning blend, and bring to a boil. Gradually add kale, a few handfuls at a time, stirring to let it wilt down. Add baked tofu, cover, reduce heat, and simmer for 15 minutes or until kale is tender. Stir in lime juice and top with sliced scallions.

PER SERVING: CALORIES 397; PROTEIN 18g; CARBOHYDRATES 41g; TOTAL FAT 19g; SATURATED FAT 2.9g; SODIUM 158mg; FIBER 6g; BETA-CAROTENE 11,341ug; VITAMIN C 149mg; CALCIUM 273mg; IRON 4.8mg; FOLATE 83ug; MAGNESIUM 82mg; ZINC 1.3mg; SELENIUM 13.8ug

Cremini Ratatouille

SERVES 2

INGREDIENTS

1 medium onion, thinly sliced

2 garlic cloves, chopped

1½ cups chopped tomatoes, fresh or packaged in BPA-free cartons

1 medium eggplant, cut into 1-inch dice

1 medium zucchini, sliced crosswise 1-inch thick

10 ounces cremini or other mushrooms, sliced

1 medium red pepper, cut into 1-inch pieces

1 teaspoon oregano

1 teaspoon basil

1 teaspoon Mrs. Dash Tomato Basil Garlic Seasoning or Dr. Fuhrman's MatoZest

DIRECTIONS

Heat ⅛ cup water in a large, deep skillet. Water-sauté the onion until softened, about 3 minutes. Add the garlic and cook for 1 minute, adding more water as necessary to keep from scorching. Reduce the heat to moderately low and add the tomatoes, eggplant, zucchini, mushrooms, red pepper, oregano, basil, and seasoning. Cover and cook, stirring occasionally, until vegetables are very tender, about 1 hour.

Serve warm or at room temperature.

PER SERVING: CALORIES 90; PROTEIN 7g; CARBOHYDRATES 19g; TOTAL FAT 0.9g; SATURATED FAT 0.2g; SODIUM 17mg; FIBER 7.9g; BETA-CAROTENE 863ug; VITAMIN C 61mg; CALCIUM 45mg; IRON 1.4mg; FOLATE 85ug; MAGNESIUM 49mg; ZINC 1mg; SELENIUM 7.5ug

> Mushrooms are a powerful food that enables superior immune function and strong protection against cancer. Even a small amount of mushrooms eaten daily shows this benefit.

Tofu Fillets with Mushroom Wine Sauce 🌿

SERVES 4

INGREDIENTS

16 ounces extra-firm tofu, drained

FOR THE MARINADE:

3 cloves garlic, pressed

1 tablespoon chopped shallots

1 cup low-sodium or no-salt-added vegetable broth

¼ cup balsamic vinegar

Pinch of hot pepper flakes

FOR THE MUSHROOM WINE SAUCE:

2 cloves garlic, chopped

¼ cup thinly sliced shallots

1 medium red bell pepper, seeded and sliced in thin strips

2 large portobello mushrooms, sliced

¼ pound shiitake mushrooms, sliced

¼ pound button mushrooms, sliced

½ cup red wine or low-sodium vegetable broth

½ cup chopped fresh parsley

No-salt seasoning blend, adjusted to taste, or 1 tablespoon Dr. Fuhrman's MatoZest

1 teaspoon herbes de Provence

¼ teaspoon black pepper

DIRECTIONS

Press the block of tofu between several layers of paper towels to remove excess water. Slice tofu in ½-inch slices.

Whisk together garlic, shallots, vegetable broth, and vinegar. Pour over tofu and marinate for 1 hour. Bake at 350°F for 35 minutes, or until lightly browned, turning halfway through baking.

For the mushroom wine sauce, water-sauté the garlic, shallots, and red peppers until almost tender. Add all remaining ingredients and simmer until liquid is reduced and mushrooms are tender.

Serve tofu topped with mushroom wine sauce.

PER SERVING: CALORIES 171; PROTEIN 10g; CARBOHYDRATES 29g; TOTAL FAT 3g; SATURATED FAT 0.5g; SODIUM 62mg; FIBER 2g; BETA-CAROTENE 1,178ug; VITAMIN C 53mg; CALCIUM 129mg; IRON 3.3mg; FOLATE 73ug; MAGNESIUM 53mg; ZINC 1.4mg; SELENIUM 20.6ug

Oven-"Fried" Tofu with Jicama Mango Slaw and Sweet Potato Sticks

>> Executive Chef Paul Bogardus

Portobello mushroom caps, salmon, or skinless chicken breasts can be substituted for the tofu in this recipe. If using portobello mushrooms, snip the stems off and gently scrape out the black gills with a teaspoon.

SERVES 6

INGREDIENTS

FOR THE TOFU:

Nonstick cooking spray or small amount of olive oil

½ cup unsweetened soy, hemp, or almond milk

3 drops hot red pepper sauce

½ cup Kashi Multigrain Flakes, crushed

3 tablespoons chickpea or whole-wheat flour

No-salt seasoning blend, adjusted to taste, or ¼ teaspoon Dr. Fuhrman's VegiZest

½ bunch fresh thyme, picked and chopped

2 pounds extra-firm tofu, drained and sliced into ¾-inch slices and patted dry

2 teaspoons olive oil

FOR THE JICAMA MANGO SLAW:

1 cup shredded savoy cabbage

1 cup shredded radicchio

1 cup julienned jicama

2 cups diced mango

1 cup diced watermelon

¼ cup chopped fresh parsley

1 tablespoon chopped fresh sage

1 tablespoon chopped fresh thyme

No-salt seasoning blend, adjusted to taste, or 1 teaspoon Dr. Fuhrman's VegiZest

½ teaspoon ground fennel seeds

½ cup raw cashews

½ cup unsweetened soy, hemp, or almond milk

1 tablespoon raisins

3 tablespoons red wine vinegar

½ organic lemon, juiced and zested

FOR THE SWEET POTATO STICKS:

Nonstick cooking spray or small amount of olive oil

1½ pounds sweet potatoes, washed and peeled

1 teaspoon olive oil

2 teaspoons apple cider vinegar or red wine, tarragon, or balsamic vinegar

1 tablespoon fresh thyme, stemmed and chopped

Black pepper to taste

DIRECTIONS

FOR THE TOFU:

Preheat the oven to 400°F. Spray a large baking sheet with nonstick cooking spray or wipe with a small amount of olive oil.

In a large bowl, combine the milk and pepper sauce. On a sheet of wax paper, combine cereal crumbs, flour, VegiZest or other no-salt seasoning blend, and thyme. Dip tofu into milk, then dredge in the crumb mixture, coating completely.

Place tofu on the prepared baking sheet, drizzle with olive oil, and bake for 15 minutes. Turn tofu over and bake an additional 15 minutes until lightly browned.

FOR THE JICAMA MANGO SLAW:

In a large bowl, combine cabbage, radicchio, jicama, mango, and watermelon.

In a high-powered blender, blend remaining ingredients. Pour over vegetable mixture and toss until evenly coated. Cover and refrigerate at least 1 hour (overnight preferably) to allow flavors to marry.

FOR THE SWEET POTATO STICKS:

Preheat the oven to 325°F. Spray 2 baking sheets with nonstick cooking spray or wipe with a small amount of olive oil. Place the sweet potatoes in a pot and cover with cold water. Over high heat, bring potatoes to a boil and let boil for 1 minute.

Drain potatoes and, while still hot, toss with olive oil, vinegar, and thyme. Lay evenly onto the prepared baking sheets and bake in the oven for 20 minutes, until lightly browned and tender. Season with black pepper.

PER SERVING: CALORIES 436; PROTEIN 22g; CARBOHYDRATES 56g; TOTAL FAT 14.8g; SATURATED FAT 1.6g; SODIUM 108mg; FIBER 10.3g; BETA-CAROTENE 10,473ug; VITAMIN C 50mg; CALCIUM 296mg; IRON 5.5mg; FOLATE 70ug; MAGNESIUM 203mg; ZINC 1.5mg; SELENIUM 5.6ug

Eggplant Cannelloni with Pine Nut Romesco Sauce 🌿

SERVES 6

INGREDIENTS

FOR THE EGGPLANT:

2 large eggplants, peeled and sliced lengthwise ½-inch thick

2–3 tablespoons water

2 medium red bell peppers, seeded and coarsely chopped

1 medium onion, coarsely chopped

1 cup chopped carrots

½ cup chopped celery

4 cloves garlic

8 ounces baby spinach

No-salt seasoning blend, adjusted to taste, or 1 tablespoon Dr. Fuhrman's VegiZest

1 cup cooked quinoa, Kamut, barley, spelt, or brown rice

2 cups no-salt-added or low-sodium pasta sauce

3 ounces nondairy, mozzarella-type cheese, shredded

FOR THE PINE NUT ROMESCO SAUCE:

½ cup onion, chopped

2 cloves garlic, chopped

½ tomato, chopped

1 teaspoon ancho chili powder

½ cup roasted red peppers

2 tablespoons water

2 tablespoons sherry vinegar

2 tablespoons pine nuts (see Note)

2 tablespoons nutritional yeast

DIRECTIONS

Preheat the oven to 350°F. Lightly oil a nonstick baking pan. Arrange eggplant in a single layer in the pan. Bake about 20 minutes or until eggplant is flexible enough to roll up easily. Set aside.

Heat 2 tablespoons water in a large pan, add the bell pepper, onion, carrots, celery, and garlic and sauté until just tender, adding more water if needed. Add the spinach and VegiZest or other no-salt seasoning blend, and cook until spinach is wilted. Add the cooked quinoa.

Transfer to a mixing bowl. Mix in 2–3 tablespoons of the pasta sauce and all of the shredded cheese. Spread about ¼ cup of the pasta sauce in a baking pan. Put some of the vegetable mixture on each eggplant slice, roll up, and place in the pan. Pour remaining sauce over the eggplant rolls. Bake for 20 minutes, until heated through.

To make romesco sauce, sauté the onions, garlic, and tomatoes in a little water or white wine until the onions are translucent, add chili powder, and sauté an extra minute. Put onion mixture in a high-powered blender with the remaining ingredients and puree until smooth. Serve eggplant with a drizzle of romesco sauce.

NOTE: Use Mediterranean pine nuts if available. See box on page 90.
Raw almonds may be substituted.

PER SERVING: CALORIES 315; PROTEIN 11g; CARBOHYDRATES 50g; TOTAL FAT 10.5g; SATURATED FAT 1.9g; SODIUM 288mg; FIBER 12.8g; BETA-CAROTENE 5,357ug; VITAMIN C 133mg; CALCIUM 282mg; IRON 3.1mg; FOLATE 170ug; MAGNESIUM 126mg; ZINC 1.9mg; SELENIUM 11.2ug

No-Pasta Zucchini Lasagna 🌿

SERVES 8

INGREDIENTS

FOR THE TOFU RICOTTA:

16 ounces extra-firm tofu, drained well

¼ cup nutritional yeast

2 teaspoons lemon juice

2 tablespoons minced shallots

1 clove garlic, minced

½ cup fresh basil, chopped

No-salt seasoning blend, adjusted to taste, or 2 tablespoons Dr. Fuhrman's MatoZest

1 teaspoon dried oregano

2 teaspoons ground chia seeds

Dash of black pepper

FOR THE VEGETABLES:

2 heads broccoli, coarsely chopped

4 cups sliced mixed fresh mushrooms (such as shiitake, cremini, oyster)

4 medium bell peppers (red, yellow, and/or orange), seeded and chopped

7 ounces baby spinach

FOR THE LASAGNA:

3 cups no-salt-added or low-sodium pasta sauce, divided

2–3 medium zucchini, sliced lengthwise into thin slices

Shredded fresh basil for garnish

DIRECTIONS

Preheat the oven to 350°F.

To make the tofu "ricotta," place the tofu in a bowl and mash until crumbly. Add remaining ingredients and mix until well combined and the consistency resembles ricotta cheese. Set aside.

To prepare the vegetables, sauté the broccoli, mushrooms, bell peppers, and spinach, without water, over low heat for 5 minutes or just until tender.

To assemble the lasagna, spread a thin layer of the pasta sauce on the bottom of a baking dish. Layer the zucchini slices, sautéed vegetables, and tofu "ricotta" and then spread with pasta sauce. Repeat the layers, ending with the tofu "ricotta." Spread the remaining pasta sauce on top and bake, uncovered, for approximately 45 minutes, or until hot and bubbly. Garnish with the shredded basil.

PER SERVING: CALORIES 240; PROTEIN 12g; CARBOHYDRATES 30g; TOTAL FAT 6.7g; SATURATED FAT 0.9g; SODIUM 106mg; FIBER 9.7g; BETA-CAROTENE 2,620ug; VITAMIN C 153mg; CALCIUM 177mg; IRON 4.5mg; FOLATE 321ug; MAGNESIUM 110mg; ZINC 1.9mg; SELENIUM 14ug

Sweet Potato "Lasagna" with Swiss Chard and Arugula Walnut Pesto 🌿

>> Executive Chef Martin Oswald

The sweet potato is wonderfully offset by the earthy mushrooms and rosemary. Make a large roasting pan of this lasagna for an easy and stress-free large party.

SERVES 5

INGREDIENTS

FOR THE POMEGRANATE REDUCTION:

2 cups pomegranate juice

FOR THE ARUGULA PESTO:

2 cloves garlic

½ cup walnuts

¼ cup white balsamic vinegar

½ cup water

No-salt seasoning blend, adjusted to taste, or ½ tablespoon Dr. Fuhrman's VegiZest

½ tablespoon nutritional yeast

2 cups arugula

2 cups spinach

FOR THE LASAGNA:

2 cups shiitake mushrooms, sliced thinly

1 cup onions, chopped

½ cup white wine or low-sodium or no-salt-added vegetable stock

3 sweet potatoes, sliced thinly

No-salt seasoning blend, adjusted to taste, or 2 tablespoons Dr. Fuhrman's VegiZest

2 sprigs rosemary, chopped

2 red peppers, roasted and diced

2 cups firm tofu, sliced thinly

Black pepper to taste

FOR THE SWISS CHARD:

6 large Swiss chard leaves

5 drops olive oil

1 shallot, thinly sliced

½ teaspoon chopped garlic

1 medium zucchini, sliced into matchstick-size pieces

½ cup cooked garbanzo beans (chickpeas) or canned no-salt-added or low-sodium garbanzo beans, drained

¼ cup low-sodium or no-salt-added vegetable stock

TO FINISH THE DISH:

4 tablespoons walnuts

2 tablespoons finely sliced chives

DIRECTIONS

TO MAKE THE POMEGRANATE REDUCTION:

Place the pomegranate juice in a small pan on low heat. Simmer until the juice is thickened to a consistency of molasses (about 45 minutes). Set aside.

TO MAKE THE PESTO:

Add the garlic, walnuts, vinegar, water, VegiZest or other no-salt seasoning blend, and nutritional yeast to a high-powered blender and blend at high speed. Add the arugula and spinach and blend to a chunky consistency on low speed. Set aside.

TO MAKE THE LASAGNA:

Preheat the oven to 350°F.

Sauté the mushrooms and onions in white wine or vegetable stock in a small pan and set aside. In a 2-inch-tall baking dish, start assembling the lasagna by placing a layer of sweet potatoes, overlapping the slices. Sprinkle the sweet potato slices with VegiZest or other no-salt seasoning blend, rosemary, mushrooms, and roasted red peppers. Next, layer the tofu slices on top of the mix. Repeat the process two more times to form a "lasagna." Finish with a layer of sweet potatoes and pour the vegetable stock over the mixture. Wrap lasagna with aluminum foil and bake it in the oven for 45 minutes.

FOR THE SAUTÉED SWISS CHARD:

Pull the leaves off the stems of the Swiss chard and slice the leaves into ½-inch ribbons. Dice the stems. Sauté the stems in the olive oil with the shallots and garlic on low heat, paying attention not to burn them. The shallots and Swiss chard stems will release some moisture so give it about 3 minutes and then add the zucchini, Swiss chard ribbons, garbanzo beans, and vegetable stock. Steam for 2 more minutes.

TO FINISH THE DISH:

Place the steamed Swiss chard mixture over the lasagna. Drizzle the arugula pesto and pomegranate reduction around the dish. Garnish with walnuts and chives.

PER SERVING: CALORIES 384; PROTEIN 12g; CARBOHYDRATES 59g; TOTAL FAT 13.1g; SATURATED FAT 1.3g; SODIUM 141mg; FIBER 7.8g; BETA-CAROTENE 9,671ug; VITAMIN C 87mg; CALCIUM 155mg; IRON 4.1mg; FOLATE 134ug; MAGNESIUM 123mg; ZINC 2mg; SELENIUM 11.1ug

Garden-Stuffed Vegetables 🌿

SERVES 6

INGREDIENTS

2 medium zucchini, cut in half lengthwise, seeds and some meat removed, leaving shells intact

4 large bell peppers, assorted colors, tops sliced off, seeds removed

2 medium portobello mushrooms, stems removed

½ cup quinoa, rinsed well

1 small red bell pepper, chopped

½ pound shiitake mushrooms, chopped

3 whole green onions, chopped

2 stalks celery, chopped

1 stalk broccoli, chopped in small pieces

4 cloves garlic, chopped in small pieces

1 cup cooked lentils* or canned, no-salt-added or low-sodium lentils, drained

½ cup walnuts, coarsely chopped

2 ounces nondairy, mozzarella-type cheese, shredded

½ cup raisins (reduce to ¼ cup for diabetic or weight-loss diets)

¼ cup plus 2 tablespoons parsley, chopped, divided

2 teaspoons Bragg Liquid Aminos

No-salt seasoning blend, adjusted to taste, or 1 tablespoon Dr. Fuhrman's MatoZest

2 cups low-sodium or no-salt-added pasta sauce

Salad greens

1 tablespoon champagne vinegar

* Use ⅓ cup dry lentils; see bean cooking instructions on page 19.

DIRECTIONS

Preheat the oven to 350°F.

On a baking sheet, bake the zucchini and peppers for 5 minutes. Add portobello mushrooms and bake for an additional 15 minutes. Set aside.

Rinse the quinoa by placing in a fine-mesh strainer and running water over it. Place the quinoa in a saucepot with 1 cup water. Bring to a boil, cover, reduce heat, and let simmer for 13 to 15 minutes, until all the water is absorbed. Set aside.

In a small amount of water, sauté red pepper, shiitake mushrooms, green onions, celery, broccoli, and garlic until tender and until all the water has cooked off.

In a large bowl, mix cooked quinoa, lentils, walnuts, cheese substitute, raisins, and ¼ cup chopped parsley with sautéed ingredients and season with liquid aminos and MatoZest or other no-salt seasoning blend.

Fill zucchini, mushrooms, and peppers with quinoa mixture and place in a baking dish.

Spoon pasta sauce over vegetables. Bake for 20 to 30 minutes until hot.

Serve on a bed of salad greens that have been lightly tossed with champagne vinegar.

Garnish vegetables with remaining chopped parsley.

PER SERVING: CALORIES 334; PROTEIN 15g; CARBOHYDRATES 53g; TOTAL FAT 9.7g; SATURATED FAT 1.3g; CHOLESTEROL 0.1mg; SODIUM 217mg; FIBER 11.8g; BETA-CAROTENE 2,459ug; VITAMIN C 191mg; CALCIUM 193mg; IRON 5.8mg; FOLATE 269ug; MAGNESIUM 134mg; ZINC 3mg; SELENIUM 10.3ug

Sicilian Stuffed Peppers 🌿

SERVES 3

INGREDIENTS

- ½ cup dry quinoa
- 3 large bell peppers, cut in half lengthwise, seeds and membranes removed
- 3 cloves garlic, minced
- 1 medium onion, minced
- 1 medium eggplant, diced
- 1 medium zucchini, diced
- 8 ounces mushrooms, diced
- 1½ cups low-sodium or no-salt-added tomato sauce
- 1 teaspoon dried oregano
- 2 tablespoons fresh basil

DIRECTIONS

Preheat the oven to 350°F (optional).

Place quinoa in a fine-mesh sieve and rinse under cold water for a few seconds.

In a saucepan, bring 1 cup water to a boil, add quinoa, turn down the heat to low, cover, and simmer gently until all the liquid is absorbed, about 15 minutes. Set aside.

Steam bell peppers, cut side down, over ½ inch boiling water until nearly tender, about 8 to 10 minutes.

Heat ⅛ cup water and sauté the garlic and onion. Add the eggplant, zucchini, and mushrooms and cook until eggplant and zucchini are soft. Add the cooked quinoa, tomato sauce, oregano, and basil. Spoon vegetable/quinoa mixture into peppers.

Serve immediately or bake for 15 minutes if desired.

PER SERVING: CALORIES 254; PROTEIN 12g; CARBOHYDRATES 53g; TOTAL FAT 2.8g; SATURATED FAT 0.4g; SODIUM 77mg; FIBER 14.8g; BETA-CAROTENE 2,117ug; VITAMIN C 182mg; CALCIUM 98mg; IRON 4.9mg; FOLATE 149ug; MAGNESIUM 124mg; ZINC 2.2mg; SELENIUM 8.5ug

Thanksgiving Nonmeat Loaf 🌿

SERVES 6

INGREDIENTS

- 2 tablespoons arrowroot powder
- 4 tablespoons water
- 2 teaspoons Bragg Liquid Aminos
- 1 box soft tofu, drained and patted dry with paper towel
- ¾ cup chopped walnuts
- 1¼ cups chopped onions
- ½ cup chopped organic celery
- 2 cups chopped portobello mushrooms
- 1 tablespoon water
- No-salt seasoning blend, adjusted to taste, or 1 tablespoon Dr. Fuhrman's MatoZest
- 2 teaspoons Spike (no salt)
- 1 teaspoon dried oregano
- 1½ teaspoons dried basil
- ½ teaspoon dried sage
- ¾ cup whole-grain bread crumbs
- 1½ cups cooked brown rice

DIRECTIONS

Preheat the oven to 350°F.

Mix arrowroot powder, water, aminos, and tofu together in a high-powered blender. Add walnuts and blend until smooth.

Sauté onions, celery, and mushrooms in water with seasonings and herbs until vegetables are soft, stirring occasionally.

In a bowl, mix together tofu mixture, vegetables, bread crumbs, and cooked rice.

Using a paper towel, spread a small amount of olive oil in a loaf pan. Add mixture to pan and bake for 1 hour and 15 minutes. Let cool for 30 minutes. Turn loaf out and slice.

NOTE: May be served with low-sodium ketchup and thinly sliced raw onion.

PER SERVING: CALORIES 350; PROTEIN 15g; CARBOHYDRATES 47g; TOTAL FAT 13.3g; SATURATED FAT 1.5g; CHOLESTEROL 0.2mg; SODIUM 359mg; FIBER 5.3g; BETA-CAROTENE 70ug; VITAMIN C 4mg; CALCIUM 143mg; IRON 3.1mg; FOLATE 107ug; MAGNESIUM 96mg; ZINC 3mg; SELENIUM 14.2ug

Artichoke Lentil Loaf 🌿

>> Chef Christine Waltermyer

SERVES 6

INGREDIENTS

½ cup onion, diced

6 cloves garlic, minced

3 cups mushrooms, finely chopped

¼ cup diced celery

2 tablespoons minced parsley

1 teaspoon poultry seasoning

1½ cups cooked lentils* or
1 (15-ounce) can low-sodium or
no-salt-added lentils, drained

4 artichokes, halved and steamed
(see next page) or 6 frozen artichoke
hearts, thawed and mashed

⅓ cup raw pecans, chopped finely

¼ cup rolled oats

¼ cup low-sodium ketchup (plus extra
for top of loaf), or tomato paste

2 tablespoons lemon juice

2 tablespoons arrowroot powder
(or whole-wheat flour)

No-salt seasoning blend, adjusted to
taste, or 2 tablespoons Dr. Fuhrman's
MatoZest

Freshly ground black pepper to taste

* Use ½ cup dried lentils; see bean
cooking instructions on page 19.

DIRECTIONS

Preheat the oven to 350°F.

In a sauté pan, heat 1 tablespoon water or vegetable broth. Add onion and garlic and sauté for 5 minutes. Add mushrooms, cover, and cook until mushrooms are tender. Add celery, parsley, and poultry seasoning. Sauté another 5 minutes, adding more water if needed to prevent sticking.

Place the sautéed vegetables in a bowl and add the lentils and remaining ingredients. Stir well to combine.

Lightly rub a loaf pan with a minimal amount of oil. Fill the loaf with lentil mixture and press down evenly. Spread a ⅛-inch layer of low-sodium ketchup or tomato paste over top. Bake for 1 hour. Remove from the oven and let stand at room temperature for 30 minutes before slicing and serving.

PER SERVING: CALORIES 189; PROTEIN 9g; CARBOHYDRATES 29g; TOTAL FAT 5.3g; SATURATED FAT 0.5g; SODIUM 146mg; FIBER 8.7g; BETA-CAROTENE 622ug; VITAMIN C 13mg; CALCIUM 51mg; IRON 3.6mg; FOLATE 130ug; MAGNESIUM 73mg; ZINC 1.7mg; SELENIUM 8.6ug

ANATOMY OF AN ARTICHOKE

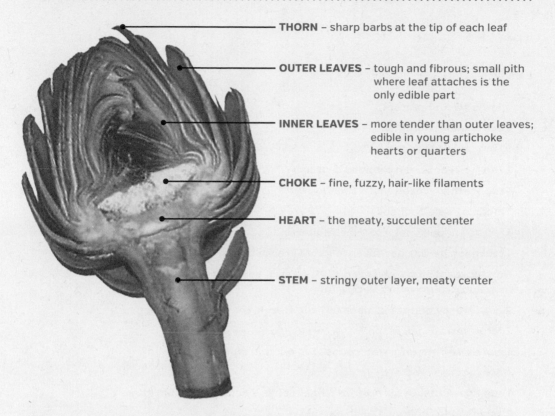

THORN – sharp barbs at the tip of each leaf

OUTER LEAVES – tough and fibrous; small pith where leaf attaches is the only edible part

INNER LEAVES – more tender than outer leaves; edible in young artichoke hearts or quarters

CHOKE – fine, fuzzy, hair-like filaments

HEART – the meaty, succulent center

STEM – stringy outer layer, meaty center

To cook artichokes, slice 1 inch off the top of each artichoke. Cut off about ¼ inch of the very bottom piece of the stem, keeping the remaining stem attached. Slice artichokes in half, lengthwise, with a small, sharp, pointed knife. Scoop out and discard the fibrous and hairy choke from the center of each half. Place the artichokes in a steamer basket over several inches of water. Bring water to a boil, cover, and steam for 18 minutes. Set artichokes aside until cool enough to handle.

To eat, peel off outer leaves one at a time. Tightly grip the outer end of the leaf, place the opposite end in your mouth, and pull through your teeth to remove the soft, pulpy, delicious portion of the leaf. You can also prepare one of my healthful dips or dressings to use as a dip. Continue until all the leaves are removed. The remaining heart can be cut into pieces and eaten.

If using in a recipe such as the Artichoke Lentil Loaf (page 204), remove the artichoke hearts and stem and transfer to a bowl. Mash lightly. Scrape off the bottom one-third of each leaf with a butter knife and add to mashed hearts and stems. Carefully scrape out the tender insides of the stems to use as well.

Vegetable Shepherd's Pie 🌿

SERVES 6

INGREDIENTS

4 large sweet potatoes

1 clove garlic, chopped

10 ounces mushrooms, sliced

1 cup fresh or frozen chopped broccoli

1 cup fresh or frozen sliced cauliflower

1 medium leek, chopped

1 red bell pepper, cut into 1-inch squares

1 teaspoon herbes de Provence (dried French herbs)

No-salt seasoning blend such as Mrs. Dash, adjusted to taste, or ¼ cup Dr. Fuhrman's VegiZest

2 cups fresh chopped spinach or 1 cup frozen, thawed and drained

2 large carrots, juiced, or ½ cup carrot juice

1 cup extra-firm tofu, water squeezed out and crumbled

4 teaspoons cornstarch

1 cup hazelnuts, Brazil nuts, or raw almonds, chopped medium-fine

2 tablespoons chopped fresh parsley

DIRECTIONS

Preheat the oven to 375°F. Bake sweet potatoes until soft, about 45 minutes. When potatoes are tender, remove to a bowl and mash. Set aside.

Heat 2 tablespoons water in a large sauté pan, add garlic and mushrooms, and sauté until mushrooms lose their water and begin to lightly brown, about 5 minutes. Remove from pan and set aside.

Place broccoli, cauliflower, leeks, bell peppers, herbes de Provence, and Dr. Fuhrman's VegiZest or other no-salt seasoning blend, in sauté pan along with 2 cups water. Simmer until almost tender, about 10 minutes. (If using frozen broccoli and cauliflower, reduce water to 1½ cups.) Add spinach and toss.

Drain and remove vegetables, reserving vegetable liquid in pot. Whisk cornstarch into carrot juice and whisk into boiling vegetable liquid until it thickens. Add sautéed mushrooms, vegetables, and crumbled tofu to sauce and toss to combine.

Divide mixture into two 8-inch pie pans. Top each with ¼ cup nuts. Spread sweet potatoes over the top and sprinkle with remaining nuts.

Bake for 20 to 30 minutes until hot and nuts are light brown. Sprinkle with parsley.

NOTE: You can make this dish ahead of time and freeze, unbaked. Cover tightly with aluminum foil before freezing. Do not defrost, but bake an additional 10 to 15 minutes.

PER SERVING: CALORIES 223; PROTEIN 6g; CARBOHYDRATES 33g; TOTAL FAT 8.5g; SATURATED FAT 0.7g; SODIUM 79mg; FIBER 6.9g; BETA-CAROTENE 10,471ug; VITAMIN C 61mg; CALCIUM 130mg; IRON 2.7mg; FOLATE 92ug; MAGNESIUM 95mg; ZINC 1.2mg; SELENIUM 4.5ug

Vegetable Tagine 🌿

Although the word tagine refers to the cone-shaped cooking vessel that the dish is traditionally made in, it has also come to refer to a Moroccan-style stew.

SERVES 4

INGREDIENTS

½ cup water

1 large onion, chopped

2 carrots, chopped

1 red bell pepper, chopped

1 zucchini, diced finely

1 clove garlic, minced

½ teaspoon cinnamon

½ teaspoon turmeric

1½ cups diced tomatoes, fresh or packaged in BPA-free cartons

2 cups low-sodium or no-salt-added vegetable stock

½ cup dried apricots, soaked for 20 minutes in enough hot water to cover (reduce to ¼ cup for diabetic or weight-loss diets)

¼ cup raisins (reduce to 2 tablespoons for diabetic or weight-loss diets)

1 tablespoon lemon juice

1½ cups cooked garbanzo beans* (chickpeas) or 1 (15-ounce) can low-sodium or no-salt-added garbanzo beans, drained

2 tablespoons minced fresh cilantro or parsley

* Use ⅓ cup dried beans; see cooking instructions on page 19.

DIRECTIONS

Heat water in a saucepan over medium heat. Add onion, carrots, and red pepper. Cover pan and cook for about 5 minutes. Add zucchini, garlic, cinnamon, turmeric, tomatoes, and vegetable stock and bring to a boil. Reduce heat to low and simmer for about 25 minutes, until vegetables are tender. Drain apricots and chop, reserving soaking water. Add apricots, soaking water, raisins, lemon juice, and chickpeas to vegetable mixture and cook 5 more minutes. Stir in cilantro or parsley and serve.

PER SERVING: CALORIES 242; PROTEIN 12g; CARBOHYDRATES 48g; TOTAL FAT 2.9g; SATURATED FAT 0.5g; SODIUM 77mg; FIBER 9.8g; BETA-CAROTENE 3,816ug; VITAMIN C 63mg; CALCIUM 89mg; IRON 3.5mg FOLATE 159ug; MAGNESIUM 67mg; ZINC 1.6mg; SELENIUM 3.1ug

Spinach with Mushrooms and Leeks 🌿

SERVES 2

INGREDIENTS

- 8 ounces mushrooms, sliced
- 2 medium leeks, sliced
- 2 cloves garlic, chopped
- 10 ounces fresh spinach
- ¼ teaspoon dried thyme
- ⅛ teaspoon black pepper
- Pinch of crushed red pepper, optional
- 1 tablespoon sherry vinegar or cooking sherry
- 1 tablespoon nutritional yeast

DIRECTIONS

In a large skillet, heat 2 tablespoons water and sauté mushrooms, leeks, and garlic until tender and until water has evaporated, about 4 minutes. Add spinach, a little at a time, cooking until wilted enough to add the remaining spinach. Add thyme, black pepper, and crushed red pepper flakes, if desired. Cover and cook until spinach is wilted, about 2 minutes. Stir in vinegar and sprinkle with nutritional yeast.

PER SERVING: CALORIES 139; PROTEIN 11g; CARBOHYDRATES 26g; TOTAL FAT 1.2g; SATURATED FAT 0.2g; SODIUM 142mg; FIBER 7.3g; BETA-CAROTENE 8,869ug; VITAMIN C 54mg; CALCIUM 215mg; IRON 7.3mg; FOLATE 507ug; MAGNESIUM 159mg; ZINC 1.8mg; SELENIUM 13.3ug

Braised Kale and Squash
with Pumpkin Seeds 🌿

SERVES 6

INGREDIENTS

2 bunches kale, tough stems and center ribs removed and leaves chopped

1 medium butternut squash or small pumpkin, peeled, seeded, and cubed

2 medium red onions, coarsely chopped

6 cloves garlic, sliced

No-salt seasoning blend, adjusted to taste, or 2 tablespoons Dr. Fuhrman's VegiZest

⅔ cup water

3 tablespoons balsamic vinegar or Dr. Fuhrman's Black Fig Vinegar

1 cup raw pumpkin seeds or sunflower seeds, lightly toasted*

* Toast seeds in the oven at 300°F for 4 minutes, or until lightly toasted.

DIRECTIONS

Place kale, squash, onion, garlic, and VegiZest or other no-salt seasoning blend in a large pot with water. Cover and steam over low heat for 20 minutes or until kale and squash are tender.

Add vinegar and toss. Serve sprinkled with lightly toasted pumpkin or sunflower seeds.

PER SERVING: CALORIES 269; PROTEIN 10g; CARBOHYDRATES 36g; TOTAL FAT 12.4g; SATURATED FAT 1.3g; SODIUM 45mg; FIBER 7.4g; BETA-CAROTENE 11,669ug; VITAMIN C 97mg; CALCIUM 186mg; IRON 4mg; FOLATE 119ug; MAGNESIUM 163mg; ZINC 1.8mg; SELENIUM 16.1ug

California Creamed Kale 🌿

SERVES 4

INGREDIENTS

- 2 bunches kale, tough stems and center ribs removed and leaves chopped
- 1 cup raw cashews
- ¾ cup unsweetened soy, hemp, or almond milk
- 4 tablespoons onion flakes
- No-salt seasoning blend, adjusted to taste, or 1 tablespoon Dr. Fuhrman's VegiZest

DIRECTIONS

Place kale in a large steamer pot. Steam 8 minutes.

Meanwhile, place remaining ingredients in a high-powered blender and blend until smooth.

Place kale in a colander and press with a clean dish towel to remove some of the excess water. In a bowl, coarsely chop and mix kale with the cream sauce.

NOTE: Sauce may also be used with broccoli, spinach, or other steamed vegetables. I also like this mixed with raw chopped red onion and a little tomato sauce on top.

PER SERVING: CALORIES 269; PROTEIN 12g; CARBOHYDRATES 25g; TOTAL FAT 15.9g; SATURATED FAT 2.7g; SODIUM 78mg; FIBER 3.7g; BETA-CAROTENE 7,060ug; VITAMIN C 90mg; CALCIUM 143mg; IRON 4.3mg; FOLATE 47ug; MAGNESIUM 139mg; ZINC 2.6mg; SELENIUM 10.2ug

Creamed Forest Kale over Wild Rice 🌿

SERVES 5

INGREDIENTS

1 cup wild rice, rinsed

2 bunches kale, tough stems and center ribs removed and leaves coarsely chopped

2 cups shiitake mushrooms, sliced

1 medium onion, chopped

2 cups fresh or frozen peas

¾ cup raw cashews

¾ cup hemp, soy, or almond milk

¼ cup onion flakes

3 tablespoons raw, unhulled sesame seeds

DIRECTIONS

In a saucepan, bring wild rice and 4 cups water to boiling. Reduce heat and simmer, covered, 50 to 60 minutes or just until kernels puff open. Remove cover, stir, cover, and let sit for 15 minutes.

In a large, covered skillet, water-sauté the kale, mushrooms, onion, and peas over medium heat, until kale is tender, about 10 minutes. Stir occasionally and add water as needed.

Meanwhile, blend the cashews, milk, and onion flakes in a food processor or high-powered blender until smooth and creamy.

Stir cashew cream sauce into kale mixture.

Serve over wild rice, topped with sesame seeds.

PER SERVING: CALORIES 338; PROTEIN 15g; CARBOHYDRATES 44g; TOTAL FAT 13.9g; SATURATED FAT 2.5g; SODIUM 118mg; FIBER 7.6g; BETA-CAROTENE 6,071ug; VITAMIN C 84mg; CALCIUM 183mg; IRON 5mg; FOLATE 106ug; MAGNESIUM 145mg; ZINC 3.6mg; SELENIUM 10.3ug

Great Greens 🌿

SERVES 4

INGREDIENTS

- 1 large bunch kale, tough stems and center ribs removed and leaves chopped
- 1 bunch Swiss chard, tough stems removed and leaves chopped
- 1 tablespoon flavored vinegar or Dr. Fuhrman's Spicy Pecan Vinegar
- 1 clove garlic, minced
- No-salt seasoning blend, adjusted to taste, or ½ tablespoon Dr. Fuhrman's VegiZest
- 1 teaspoon dried dill
- 1 teaspoon dried basil
- Black pepper to taste
- ¼ cup raw chopped pecans, lightly toasted

DIRECTIONS

Steam the kale and Swiss chard for 7 minutes. Transfer to a bowl.

Combine the remaining ingredients and add to the greens. If desired, add 2–3 tablespoons of the steaming water to adjust consistency. Serve topped with toasted pecans.

PER SERVING: CALORIES 46; PROTEIN 3g; CARBOHYDRATES 9g; TOTAL FAT 0.5g; SATURATED FAT 0.1g; SODIUM 150mg; FIBER 2.2g; BETA-CAROTENE 7,435ug; VITAMIN C 86mg; CALCIUM 117mg; IRON 2.3mg; FOLATE 25ug; MAGNESIUM 68mg; ZINC 0.5mg; SELENIUM 1.1ug

Orange Zest Chard 🌿

» Executive Chef Martin Oswald

SERVES 4

INGREDIENTS

. . . .

2 shallots, diced

2 cloves garlic, diced

2 bunches Swiss chard, stems and leaves separated and diced

1 organic orange, zested (see box on page 217) and juiced

Pinch of allspice

Pinch of chipotle chili flakes

2 tablespoons Dr. Fuhrman's Blood Orange Vinegar

DIRECTIONS

. . . .

Sauté the shallots, garlic and Swiss chard stems in a hot, dry stainless steel pan for 3 to 5 minutes, stirring constantly. Add the orange zest and juice, allspice and chipotle chili flakes. Deglaze the pan with vinegar, add the chard leaves, and steam for 3 more minutes.

. . . .

PER SERVING: CALORIES 35; PROTEIN 2g; CARBOHYDRATES 7g; TOTAL FAT 0.2g; SODIUM 156mg; FIBER 1.2g; BETA-CAROTENE 2,631ug; VITAMIN C 31mg; CALCIUM 46mg; IRON 1.5mg; FOLATE 18ug; MAGNESIUM 63mg; ZINC 0.3mg; SELENIUM 1ug

Swiss Chard and Beans Italiano 🌿

SERVES 4

INGREDIENTS

....

1 pound Swiss chard

6 garlic cloves, minced

1½ cups no-salt-added or low-sodium tomato sauce

3 plum tomatoes, chopped

1½ cups red kidney beans* or 1 (15-ounce) can low-sodium or no-salt-added kidney beans, drained

½ teaspoon no-salt Italian seasoning blend

* Use ½ cup dried beans; see cooking instructions on page 19.

DIRECTIONS

....

Combine all ingredients in a pot and simmer on low heat until chard is soft, stirring occasionally.

....

PER SERVING: CALORIES 174; PROTEIN 13g; CARBOHYDRATES 34g; TOTAL FAT 1g; SATURATED FAT 0.1g; SODIUM 262mg; FIBER 9.8g; BETA-CAROTENE 4,804ug; VITAMIN C 64mg; CALCIUM 111mg; IRON 5.3mg; FOLATE 127ug; MAGNESIUM 156mg; ZINC 1.6mg; SELENIUM 3.2ug

Brussels Sprouts with Orange and Walnuts 🍃

SERVES 4

INGREDIENTS

1 pound brussels sprouts

½ cup freshly squeezed orange juice

¼ cup walnuts

1 teaspoon organic orange zest (see box on page 217)

Freshly ground pepper to taste

DIRECTIONS

Place brussels sprouts in a steamer basket over boiling water. Cover and steam about 20 minutes or until tender.

Place steamed brussels sprouts and orange juice in a large skillet, bring to a simmer, and cook for 3 minutes. Remove from heat. Toast walnuts in a small skillet over medium heat for 2 to 3 minutes until lightly toasted. Add toasted walnuts and grated orange peel and gently toss. Season with pepper.

PER SERVING: CALORIES 111; PROTEIN 5g; CARBOHYDRATES 15g; TOTAL FAT 5.2g; SATURATED FAT 0.5g; SODIUM 29mg; FIBER 4.9g; BETA-CAROTENE 521ug; VITAMIN C 113mg; CALCIUM 59mg; IRON 1.9mg; FOLATE 86ug; MAGNESIUM 41mg; ZINC 0.7mg; SELENIUM 2.2ug

Brussels Sprouts with Butternut Squash and Currants

>> Executive Chef Martin Oswald

SERVES 4

INGREDIENTS

½ cup shallots, cut in half

2 cups brussels sprouts, leaves separated from the hearts

½ cup butternut squash, diced

½ teaspoon fresh thyme, chopped

½ organic lemon, zest only (see box)

1 tablespoon balsamic vinegar or Dr. Fuhrman's Black Fig Vinegar

2 tablespoons dried currants

2 tablespoons hemp seeds

DIRECTIONS

Preheat the oven to 350°F. Wrap the shallots and 2 tablespoons water in aluminum foil and bake for 50 minutes.

In a stainless steel pan, steam the brussels sprout hearts and butternut squash in ¼ cup water for 5 minutes. Add the shallots, thyme, brussels sprout leaves, lemon zest, vinegar, and currants. Steam 3 more minutes.

Sprinkle with hemp seeds to garnish.

PER SERVING: CALORIES 75; PROTEIN 3g; CARBOHYDRATES 14g; TOTAL FAT 1.7g; SATURATED FAT 0.2g; SODIUM 16mg; FIBER 3.1g; BETA-CAROTENE 940ug; VITAMIN C 43mg; CALCIUM 45mg; IRON 1.2mg; FOLATE 41ug; MAGNESIUM 35mg; ZINC 0.5mg; SELENIUM 1.9ug

The zest of a lemon or other citrus fruit is the outermost, colored skin that contains flavorful oils. Use a grater to take off just the colored part, not the white pith. Thoroughly washed organic oranges, lemons, or limes should be used for zesting. Dried, grated orange or lemon zest is also available in the spice section of most stores.

Broccoli Fra Diavlo 🌿

SERVES 2

INGREDIENTS

- 5 cups fresh broccoli florets
- 4 cloves garlic, chopped
- 1½ cups diced fresh tomatoes or 1 (15-ounce) can no-salt-added diced tomatoes
- 1 cup low-sodium or no-salt-added tomato or pasta sauce
- 1–2 teaspoons Italian seasoning
- Dash of dried hot pepper flakes
- ¼ cup nutritional yeast
- ½ teaspoon Spanish paprika

DIRECTIONS

Steam broccoli until tender.

In a large saucepan over medium heat, sauté garlic in ¼ cup water for 3 to 4 minutes. Add tomatoes, tomato sauce, Italian seasoning, and hot pepper flakes to taste. Simmer 10 minutes.

Stir in broccoli, nutritional yeast, and Spanish paprika.

PER SERVING: CALORIES 209; PROTEIN 19g; CARBOHYDRATES 38g; TOTAL FAT 1.5g; SATURATED FAT 0.2g; SODIUM 116mg; FIBER 15g; BETA-CAROTENE 1,712ug; VITAMIN C 238mg; CALCIUM 194mg; IRON 6.2mg; FOLATE 803ug; MAGNESIUM 126mg; ZINC 2.8mg; SELENIUM 7.3ug

Cauliflower and Green Pea Curry 🌿

SERVES 4

INGREDIENTS

- 3 garlic cloves, minced
- 1 medium onion, chopped
- 1 small carrot, grated
- 2 teaspoons minced fresh ginger
- 1 tablespoon curry powder
- 1 teaspoon ground cumin
- 1 head cauliflower, cut into florets
- 1½ cups chopped tomatoes, fresh or packaged in BPA-free containers
- 1 cup fresh or frozen green peas
- ¼ cup water
- 1 tablespoon fresh lemon juice

DIRECTIONS

Water-sauté garlic, onion, and carrots until tender. Add ginger, curry powder, and cumin and sauté an additional minute. Add cauliflower, tomatoes, peas, and water. Cover and simmer for 7 minutes or until cauliflower is tender, adding more water if needed to adjust consistency.

Stir in lemon juice.

PER SERVING: CALORIES 107; PROTEIN 8g; CARBOHYDRATES 22g; TOTAL FAT 0.8g; SATURATED FAT 0.1g; SODIUM 103mg; FIBER 7.7g; BETA-CAROTENE 2,029ug; VITAMIN C 90mg; CALCIUM 76mg; IRON 2mg; FOLATE 126ug; MAGNESIUM 49mg; ZINC 1mg; SELENIUM 2.3ug

Cauliflower Spinach Mashed "Potatoes" 🌿

SERVES 4

INGREDIENTS

- 6 cups cauliflower florets, fresh or frozen
- 4 cloves garlic, sliced
- 10 ounces fresh spinach
- ½ cup raw cashew butter
- Soy, almond, or hemp milk, if needed to thin
- No-salt seasoning blend, adjusted to taste, or 2 tablespoons Dr. Fuhrman's VegiZest
- ¼ teaspoon nutmeg

DIRECTIONS

Steam cauliflower and garlic about 8 to 10 minutes or until tender. Drain and press out as much water as possible in strainer.

Place spinach in steamer, steam until just wilted, and set aside.

Process cauliflower, garlic, and cashew butter in a food processor until creamy and smooth. If necessary, add soy milk to adjust consistency.

Add VegiZest or other no-salt seasoning blend and nutmeg. Mix in wilted spinach.

PER SERVING: CALORIES 164; PROTEIN 9g; CARBOHYDRATES 18g; TOTAL FAT 8.5g; SATURATED FAT 1.7g; SODIUM 124mg; FIBER 5.7g; BETA-CAROTENE 4,599ug; VITAMIN C 93mg; CALCIUM 116mg; IRON 3.8mg; FOLATE 234ug; MAGNESIUM 121mg; ZINC 1.7mg; SELENIUM 3.9ug

Lemon Cauliflower Risotto 🌿

» Executive Chef Martin Oswald

SERVES 4

INGREDIENTS

½ onion, diced

2 cloves garlic, finely chopped

½ cup low-sodium or no-salt-added vegetable broth

6 cups finely chopped cauliflower florets (tops of florets only, no stems)

½ organic lemon, juiced and zested (see box on page 217)

1 cup roasted red bell peppers, sliced

1 tablespoon nutritional yeast

2 cups spinach, finely sliced

4 tablespoons raw almond butter

2 tablespoons raw almonds, chopped

2 tablespoons sliced chives, divided

DIRECTIONS

Sauté the onion and garlic in a stainless pot without water, stirring often until golden brown, about 7 minutes.

Add the vegetable broth and cauliflower and sauté for 3 minutes. Add all other ingredients, except the almonds and 1 tablespoon chives, and cook for 3 more minutes or until cauliflower is al dente. Sprinkle the almonds and remaining chives over the risotto.

PER SERVING: CALORIES 209; PROTEIN 9g; CARBOHYDRATES 21g; TOTAL FAT 12.5g; SATURATED FAT 1.3g; CHOLESTEROL 2.1mg; SODIUM 73mg; FIBER 6.4g; BETA-CAROTENE 1,861ug; VITAMIN C 132mg; CALCIUM 114mg; IRON 2.2mg; FOLATE 155ug; MAGNESIUM 103mg; ZINC 1.5mg; SELENIUM 3.1ug

"Cheesy" Barley Risotto 🌿

» Talia Fuhrman

SERVES 4

INGREDIENTS

- 1 teaspoon olive oil
- 1 cup hulled barley (see Note)
- 1 teaspoon dried oregano
- 1 teaspoon basil
- 1 clove garlic, minced
- ½ large onion, thinly sliced
- 1½ cups diced tomatoes, fresh or packaged in BPA-free containers
- 1 cup unsweetened soy, hemp, or almond milk
- 2 tablespoons water, plus more if needed
- ½ cup nutritional yeast
- ½ tablespoon miso, mixed with ½ tablespoon water
- 1 cup thinly sliced shiitake mushrooms
- ¼ cup unsulfured, no-salt-added dried tomatoes, finely chopped
- 2 cups frozen spinach, thawed, or 6 cups fresh spinach
- No-salt Italian seasoning blend, adjusted to taste, or 2 tablespoons Dr. Fuhrman's MatoZest

DIRECTIONS

Place olive oil and 2 tablespoons water in a medium pot along with barley, oregano, and basil. Over medium heat, stir the barley until it is well coated with the oil and water. When the barley begins to simmer, add the minced garlic and onion. Reduce heat to low-medium and cook for 1 minute.

Stir in the diced tomatoes, milk, water, nutritional yeast, and miso. Bring to a boil, reduce heat to low, cover, and cook (allowing a bit of air to escape) for 15 minutes.

Add shiitake mushrooms, dried tomatoes, spinach, and MatoZest or other no-salt Italian seasoning blend. Cook for another 15 to 20 minutes or until desired consistency, stirring every 5 minutes or so, being careful not to burn the barley on the bottom of the pot.

The mixture should be creamy, not soupy, and the barley will be chewy and not mushy. Serve immediately.

NOTE: Hulled barley, also known as barley groats, is the whole-grain form of barley. Pearl barley may also be used but it is lower in nutritional value. Pearl barley undergoes extensive processing that removes the outer hulls along with the bran. Hulled barley has only the outer layer removed, leaving the bran layer intact. Most recipes call for pearl barley or intend for cooks to use this type even if they don't specify. However, it is usually fine to substitute hulled barley. Just be aware that you may need to adjust the cooking time.

Hulled barley can take 2 hours to cook to a soft and mushy texture, but, after just 35 minutes, it is chewy and ready to eat. If you don't want it as chewy, cook longer, adding more water if needed, until it reaches desired texture.

PER SERVING: CALORIES 371; PROTEIN 26g; CARBOHYDRATES 66g; TOTAL FAT 5.5g; SATURATED FAT 0.8g; SODIUM 354mg; FIBER 19.3g; BETA-CAROTENE 6,687ug; VITAMIN C 34mg; CALCIUM 208mg; IRON 9.6mg; FOLATE 708ug; MAGNESIUM 186mg; ZINC 4.2mg; SELENIUM 40.6ug

Green Beans in a Cloud 🌿

SERVES 3

INGREDIENTS

4 cups cut fresh green beans

⅛ cup water

1½ tablespoons raw cashew butter

1 teaspoon no-salt-added stone-ground mustard

1 clove garlic, minced

1 tablespoon finely chopped onion

1 teaspoon lemon juice

Freshly ground black pepper to taste

DIRECTIONS

Steam green beans for 8 minutes or until crisp-tender.

Mash the water and cashew butter together with a fork to thin, and then whisk in remaining ingredients and toss with steamed green beans.

PER SERVING: CALORIES 101; PROTEIN 5g; CARBOHYDRATES 14g; TOTAL FAT 4.2g; SATURATED FAT 0.8g; SODIUM 39mg; FIBER 5.3g; BETA-CAROTENE 823ug; VITAMIN C 26mg; CALCIUM 62mg; IRON 2.1mg; FOLATE 61ug; MAGNESIUM 59mg; ZINC 0.8mg; SELENIUM 2.5ug

Summer Corn and Tomato Sauté 🌿

SERVES 4

INGREDIENTS

- 2 cups fresh, raw corn kernels
- ¼ cup chopped red onion
- 1 pound tomatoes, chopped
- ¼ cup chopped fresh basil
- Freshly ground black pepper to taste

DIRECTIONS

Heat 2 tablespoons water in a skillet and sauté corn and onion, stirring occasionally until corn is tender, about 5 minutes. Remove from heat and let stand for 5 minutes. Stir in tomatoes and basil and season with black pepper.

PER SERVING: CALORIES 96; PROTEIN 6g; CARBOHYDRATES 22g; TOTAL FAT 0.9g; SATURATED FAT 0.1g; SODIUM 8mg; FIBER 3.5g; BETA-CAROTENE 594ug; VITAMIN C 21mg; CALCIUM 20mg; IRON 0.7mg; FOLATE 50ug; MAGNESIUM 30mg; ZINC 0.5mg; SELENIUM 0.6ug

Mushroom Stroganoff 🌿

Delicious served over smashed steamed cauliflower, parsnips, or baked potato or on a bed of steamed kale or spinach.

SERVES 4

INGREDIENTS

- 1 medium onion, chopped
- 1 clove garlic, minced
- 1 pound mushrooms, thinly sliced
- 2 tablespoons fresh lemon juice
- 1 tablespoon fresh tarragon, chopped, or 1 teaspoon dried tarragon
- 1 tablespoon sweet paprika
- 1 cup low-sodium or no-salt-added vegetable broth
- 3 tablespoons tahini (or 3 tablespoons unhulled sesame seeds pureed with ¼ cup water)

DIRECTIONS

In a nonstick skillet, water-sauté onion and garlic until soft. Add mushrooms and continue cooking until mushrooms soften and lose their moisture. Add lemon juice, tarragon, and paprika and mix well.

Blend vegetable broth and tahini. (Heating the broth makes blending easier.)

Pour over mushroom mixture and mix well. Simmer until mixture thickens slightly or until desired consistency.

PER SERVING: CALORIES 123; PROTEIN 7g; CARBOHYDRATES 12g; TOTAL FAT 7g; SATURATED FAT 1g; SODIUM 30mg; FIBER 2.8g; BETA-CAROTENE 436ug; VITAMIN C 10mg; CALCIUM 46mg; IRON 2mg; FOLATE 40ug; MAGNESIUM 32mg; ZINC 1.3mg; SELENIUM 11ug

Mushroom-Stuffed Cabbage Rolls 🌿

SERVES 4

INGREDIENTS

2 cups chopped mushrooms

1 cup diced zucchini

¾ cup chopped red bell pepper

¾ cup chopped onion

1 cup cooked wild rice (see Note)

⅓ cup raisins (reduce to 2 tablespoons for diabetic or weight-loss diets)

¼ cup walnuts, chopped

1 teaspoon dried basil

½ teaspoon dried marjoram

½ teaspoon dried thyme

½ teaspoon Mrs. Dash tomato-flavor seasoning or 1 teaspoon Dr. Fuhrman's MatoZest

1 large head cabbage

2 cups no-salt-added or low-sodium tomato sauce

DIRECTIONS

Preheat the oven to 350°F.

In a large saucepan, heat 2 tablespoons water and water-sauté mushrooms, zucchini, red pepper, and onion until tender. Add cooked wild rice, raisins, walnuts, basil, marjoram, thyme, and MatoZest or Mrs. Dash tomato-flavor seasoning.

Meanwhile, cook cabbage in boiling water until leaves fall off head. Set aside 8 large leaves (refrigerate remaining cabbage for another use). Cut out the thick vein from each leaf. Overlap cut ends before filling.

Spoon ¼ to ½ cup mushroom/rice mixture onto the thick bottom of each cabbage leaf. Roll the leaf over once, then fold the 2 sides in and finish rolling.

Cover the bottom of a casserole dish with some of the tomato sauce. Place rolls in the casserole, seam-side down. Pour remaining sauce over rolls, covering cabbage completely. Bake until cabbage is cooked and rolls are heated through, about 30 minutes.

NOTE: Wild rice cooking tip: Rinse rice. Combine 1 cup wild rice and 4 cups water in a heavy saucepan. Bring to a boil, cover, and simmer over low heat for 45 minutes, until rice has opened and fluffed out. Remove cover, stir, cover, and let sit for 15 minutes. Drain any excess water. One cup uncooked wild rice yields 3–4 cups cooked wild rice.

PER SERVING: CALORIES 231; PROTEIN 9g; CARBOHYDRATES 42g; TOTAL FAT 5.9g; SATURATED FAT 0.7g; SODIUM 671mg; FIBER 8.4g; BETA-CAROTENE 795ug; VITAMIN C 94mg; CALCIUM 96mg; IRON 3mg; FOLATE 107ug; MAGNESIUM 86mg; ZINC 1.5mg; SELENIUM 10.5ug

Portobello Mushrooms and Beans

SERVES 2

INGREDIENTS

1 large onion, chopped

2 garlic cloves, chopped

2 large portobello mushroom caps, thinly sliced

½ cup red wine (or low-sodium vegetable broth)

1 large tomato, diced, or 8 cherry tomatoes, halved

1½ cups cooked garbanzo beans* (chickpeas) or 1 (15-ounce) can no-salt-added
or low-sodium garbanzo beans, drained

* Use ½ cup dried beans; see cooking instructions on page 19.

DIRECTIONS

Water-sauté the onion and garlic for 2 minutes or until onions are soft. Add the
mushrooms and the red wine (or broth) and continue cooking for 5 minutes, until
mushrooms are tender. Add the tomatoes and garbanzo beans. Simmer for 5 minutes.

PER SERVING: CALORIES 143; PROTEIN 11g; CARBOHYDRATES 25g; TOTAL FAT 2.1g; SATURATED FAT 0.3g; SODIUM 21mg;
FIBER 6.6g; BETA-CAROTENE 414ug; VITAMIN C 15mg; CALCIUM 50mg; IRON 2.3mg; FOLATE 130ug; MAGNESIUM 46mg; ZINC 1.4mg;
SELENIUM 6ug

To add some zest to your dishes without adding salt,
try making a seasoning blend called Gremolata.
Toss together:
1–2 cloves garlic, finely minced
¼ cup fresh, flat-leaf parsley, minced
2 teaspoons grated lemon zest (use organic lemon)

This mixture can be sprinkled over
vegetable dishes, soups, or sautéed mushrooms just before serving.
May also be served at the table as a condiment.

Spinach-Stuffed Mushrooms 🌿

SERVES 3

INGREDIENTS

1 small onion, chopped

12 large mushrooms, stems separated and chopped

1 clove garlic, minced

½ teaspoon dried thyme

¼ cup low-sodium or no-salt-added vegetable broth

5 ounces fresh spinach

2 tablespoons raw almond butter

1 tablespoon nutritional yeast

¼ teaspoon black pepper, or to taste

DIRECTIONS

Preheat the oven to 350°F.

In a large pan, heat 2–3 tablespoons of water and water-sauté chopped onion for 2 minutes, add mushroom stems, garlic, and thyme and continue to sauté until onions and mushrooms are tender, about 3 minutes. Add mushroom caps to the pan, along with vegetable broth, bring to a simmer, and cook for 5 minutes.

Remove mushroom caps from pan and place on a lightly oiled baking sheet. Add spinach to onion mixture remaining in pan and heat until wilted. Remove from heat and stir in almond butter, nutritional yeast, and black pepper.

Fill mushroom caps with spinach/onion mixture and bake for 15 to 20 minutes or until golden brown.

PER SERVING: CALORIES 121; PROTEIN 7g; CARBOHYDRATES 12g; TOTAL FAT 6.8g; SATURATED FAT 0.7g; SODIUM 53mg; FIBER 3.8g; BETA-CAROTENE 2,664ug; VITAMIN C 18mg; CALCIUM 99mg; IRON 3mg; FOLATE 222ug; MAGNESIUM 86mg; ZINC 1.3mg; SELENIUM 7.5ug

Polenta with Wilted Greens, Roasted Portobello Mushrooms, and Black Cherry Vinaigrette 🌿

» Chef James Rohrbacher

During pomegranate season, use Dr. Fuhrman's Pomegranate Balsamic Vinegar instead of the Black Cherry Vinegar and substitute 1 cup pomegranate seeds for the cherries.

SERVES 4

INGREDIENTS

FOR THE BLACK CHERRY VINAIGRETTE:

½ cup Dr. Fuhrman's Black Cherry Vinegar

1 cup water

2 teaspoons arrowroot powder, dissolved in ¼ cup cold water

FOR THE POLENTA:

4 portobello mushrooms, cleaned and sliced into 2-inch-long slices

½ cup red wine

4 cloves garlic, roughly chopped

½ onion, diced

4 sprigs thyme

1 sprig rosemary

Freshly ground pepper to taste

3 cups water

¾ cup cornmeal

2 bunches mixed greens (kale, collard, bok choy, etc.), washed, chopped, and steamed in water or white wine for 15 minutes or until tender

1 cup pitted and chopped fresh or frozen cherries

DIRECTIONS

Preheat the oven to 375°F.

To make the black cherry vinaigrette, bring the vinegar and 1 cup water to a boil in a small saucepan. Once boiling, whisk in the arrowroot/cold water mixture and let boil for 2 minutes, but no longer, whisking occasionally. Remove from the heat and let the vinaigrette cool to room temperature.

To prepare polenta, place the mushrooms in a roasting pan, pour the wine over them, and sprinkle with the chopped garlic and onions. Lay the thyme and rosemary sprigs on top and sprinkle with freshly ground black pepper. Cover the pan with foil and bake for 45 to 60 minutes until tender. Remove the herb sprigs.

Meanwhile, bring 3 cups water to a boil over high heat. When water is boiling, slowly whisk cornmeal into the boiling water. When all the cornmeal is added, reduce heat to a very low simmer, cover, and continue cooking until the polenta is smooth and thick, about 10 to 20 minutes, stirring every 5 minutes.

For a soft polenta, stir the greens into the hot polenta and serve in individual large pasta bowls topped with the mushrooms, desired amount of the vinaigrette, and the cherries.

For a baked polenta, pour the hot cooked polenta into an 8 x 8-inch nonstick cake pan and chill until firm. Remove from the refrigerator and turn out onto a cutting board. Cut into quarters and then cut quarters into half to make triangles. Place the triangles on a nonstick baking sheet and put under the broiler until lightly browned. To serve, place the steamed greens on the bottom of a large bowl or plate. Top with 2 polenta triangles and the mushrooms, drizzle desired amount of vinaigrette, and sprinkle with cherries.

PER SERVING: CALORIES 351; PROTEIN 20g; CARBOHYDRATES 67g; TOTAL FAT 2.2g; SATURATED FAT 0.3g; SODIUM 69mg; FIBER 14.1g; BETA-CAROTENE 255ug; VITAMIN C 20mg; CALCIUM 147mg; IRON 5.9mg; FOLATE 256ug; MAGNESIUM 118mg; ZINC 4.7mg; SELENIUM 73.6ug

Acorn Squash Supreme

SERVES 2

INGREDIENTS

- 1 large acorn squash
- ¼ cup dried, unsulfured apricots, soaked, until soft, in just enough water to almost cover, then diced
- 1½ cups pineapple, chopped
- 2 tablespoons raisins
- 2 tablespoons walnuts and cashews, chopped
- ½ teaspoon Ceylon cinnamon

DIRECTIONS

Preheat the oven to 350°F.

Cut squash in half, remove seeds, and bake facedown in ½ inch of water for 45 minutes.

Meanwhile, combine the apricots and soaking liquid, pineapple, raisins, and nuts.

After the squash has cooked, scoop the fruit/nut mixture into the squash's center. Place in a pan and cover loosely with aluminum foil. Bake for an additional 30 minutes. Sprinkle with cinnamon, then put it back in the oven for 5 more minutes.

PER SERVING: CALORIES 257; PROTEIN 4g; CARBOHYDRATES 57g; TOTAL FAT 4.4g; SATURATED FAT 0.8g; SODIUM 12mg; FIBER 6.6g; BETA-CAROTENE 865ug; VITAMIN C 66mg; CALCIUM 104mg; IRON 3mg; FOLATE 62ug; MAGNESIUM 113mg; ZINC 1mg; SELENIUM 2.6ug

Sweet Potato and Asparagus Ragout 🌿

SERVES 6

INGREDIENTS

- 2 medium sweet potatoes, peeled and chopped into bite-size pieces
- 6 unsulfured, dried figs, chopped (reduce to 3 figs for diabetic or weight-loss diets)
- 12 ounces baby spinach
- 2 cups low-sodium or no-salt-added vegetable broth
- 2 large leeks, white and pale green parts only, washed thoroughly* and cut into ½-inch slices
- 1 clove garlic, minced
- 1 pound fresh asparagus, trimmed and cut diagonally into 1-inch pieces
- 7 ounces fresh shiitake mushrooms, chopped
- 2 tablespoons fresh lemon juice
- 3 tablespoons chopped fresh parsley
- 3 tablespoons chopped fresh mint leaves

* To remove dirt from leeks, split lengthwise, separate, then wash thoroughly.

DIRECTIONS

Place potatoes and figs in a steamer and steam until potatoes are tender, about 10 minutes. Add spinach on top of potatoes in the steamer, cover, and allow to wilt. Once spinach is wilted, transfer mixture to a bowl and set aside.

Add vegetable broth, leeks, garlic, and asparagus to a skillet. Cover and simmer until leeks and asparagus are tender, about 10 minutes. Remove with a slotted spoon and transfer to the bowl with potatoes and spinach.

In the same skillet, sauté mushrooms, stirring occasionally, until mushrooms are softened, about 2 minutes. Add mushrooms to potato/spinach/asparagus mixture. Add lemon juice, parsley, and mint leaves and gently toss.

PER SERVING: CALORIES 181; PROTEIN 7g; CARBOHYDRATES 37g; TOTAL FAT 2.6g; SATURATED FAT 0.6g; SODIUM 96mg; FIBER 7.6g; BETA-CAROTENE 8,009ug; VITAMIN C 31mg; CALCIUM 149mg; IRON 5mg; FOLATE 186ug; MAGNESIUM 105mg; ZINC 1.6mg; SELENIUM 67.2ug

Spaghetti Squash Primavera

SERVES 4

INGREDIENTS

1 medium spaghetti squash

1½ carrots, diagonally sliced

½ cup diagonally sliced celery

3 cloves garlic, minced

1½ cups shredded cabbage

1 small zucchini, chopped into small pieces

1½ cups cooked pinto beans* or 1 (15-ounce) can low-sodium or no-salt-added pinto beans, drained

1½ cups chopped tomatoes, fresh or packaged in BPA-free cartons

⅓ cup low-sodium or no-salt-added vegetable broth

1 teaspoon dried thyme

2 tablespoons chopped fresh parsley

1 cup low-sodium or no-salt-added pasta sauce

Nutritarian "Parmesan" (see box)

* Use ½ cup dried beans; see cooking instructions on page 19.

Nutritarian Parmesan is easy
to make and you can sprinkle it on anything.

Place ½ cup raw almonds (walnuts or pine nuts also work)
and ½ cup nutritional yeast in a food processor and pulse
until the texture of grated Parmesan is achieved. Place in an
airtight container and refrigerate. Keeps indefinitely.

DIRECTIONS

Preheat the oven to 350°F.

Slice spaghetti squash in half lengthwise and remove seeds. Place both halves upside down on a baking sheet. Bake for 45 minutes or until tender.

Meanwhile, cook carrots and celery in 2 tablespoons water in a covered pan over medium heat for 10 minutes, stirring occasionally. Add a little more water if needed. Add garlic, cabbage, and zucchini and cook, covered, for another 10 minutes. Stir in remaining ingredients, except for pasta sauce and "Parmesan." Cover and simmer for 10 minutes or until carrots are tender. When squash is done, remove from the oven and, using a fork, scrape spaghetti-like strands from squash into a bowl. Add pasta sauce and combine by mixing thoroughly.

Mix the vegetables, beans, and herbs with the squash/pasta sauce mixture and serve on a bed of shredded romaine lettuce, if desired, or place back in the hollowed-out squash bowls.

Sprinkle with nutritarian "Parmesan."

PER SERVING: CALORIES 268; PROTEIN 13g; CARBOHYDRATES 51g; TOTAL FAT 4.5g; SATURATED FAT 0.7g; SODIUM 94mg; FIBER 14.6g; BETA-CAROTENE 5,555ug; VITAMIN C 63mg; CALCIUM 158mg; IRON 4.3mg; FOLATE 291ug; MAGNESIUM 101mg; ZINC 1.7mg; SELENIUM 6.1ug

Chard and Sweet Potato Gratin 🌿

SERVES 6

INGREDIENTS

Small amount of olive oil

8 ounces tempeh, sliced as thinly as possible

1 teaspoon chopped fresh ginger

1 small onion, finely chopped

½ cup chopped green bell pepper

8 cups Swiss chard, stems removed, coarsely chopped

4 medium (about 1¼ pounds) sweet potatoes, peeled and sliced ⅛-inch thick

2 cups unsweetened hemp, soy, or almond milk

⅛ teaspoon nutmeg

⅛ teaspoon black pepper

¼ cup nondairy mozzarella-style cheese*

2 tablespoons flax seeds, toasted

* Daiya brand cheese substitute is a good choice.

DIRECTIONS

Preheat the oven to 400°F. Rub a 9x13-inch baking dish with a small amount of olive oil.

Place tempeh in a saucepan with water to cover, simmer for 10 minutes, then remove from water.

Heat ⅛ cup water in a large pan and water-sauté ginger, onion, and green pepper until softened. Add Swiss chard and cook until just tender.

Arrange one-third of the sliced sweet potatoes on the bottom of the prepared baking dish. Place one-half of the tempeh and one-half of the Swiss chard mixture on top. Arrange another one-third of the sweet potato slices, then the remaining tempeh, then the Swiss chard, followed by the remaining sweet potato.

Combine milk, nutmeg, and black pepper. Pour over dish. Cover with foil and bake for 35 minutes. Remove foil, top with nondairy mozzarella cheese, and bake for an additional 15 minutes. Sprinkle with toasted flax seeds.

PER SERVING: CALORIES 349; PROTEIN 21g; CARBOHYDRATES 46g; TOTAL FAT 11.1g; SATURATED FAT 2g; SODIUM 347mg; FIBER 8.4g; BETA-CAROTENE 14,167ug; VITAMIN C 42mg; CALCIUM 245mg; IRON 5.3mg; FOLATE 68ug; MAGNESIUM 188mg; ZINC 2.2mg; SELENIUM 9.6ug

Tempeh originated in Indonesia. It is made from fermented soybeans, sometimes mixed with grains, and formed in the shape of a patty or cake. It has a nutty taste, but easily absorbs the flavors of other foods with which it is cooked, making it adaptable to many types of dishes.

Channna Saag
(Spicy Chickpeas with Spinach) ✿

SERVES 2

INGREDIENTS

1 medium onion, thinly sliced

2 garlic cloves, crushed

1 inch piece ginger, grated

2 medium tomatoes, chopped

1 teaspoon ground coriander

1 teaspoon garam marsala (an Indian spice mixture)

1 teaspoon ground cardamom

1 teaspoon ground cinnamon

12 ounces spinach, chopped (frozen or fresh)

1½ cups cooked garbanzo beans (chickpeas)* or 1 (15-ounce) can no-salt-added or low-sodium garbanzo beans, drained

⅛ teaspoon cayenne pepper, or to taste

* Use ⅔ cup dried beans; see cooking instructions on page 19.

DIRECTIONS

Heat 2 to 3 tablespoons water in a large pan. Water-sauté onion, garlic, and ginger until tender. Add the tomatoes, spices, and spinach and cook 5 minutes. Stir in the chickpeas and cayenne pepper and cook for another 5 minutes.

PER SERVING: CALORIES 298; PROTEIN 21g; CARBOHYDRATES 53g; TOTAL FAT 4.3g; SATURATED FAT 0.5g; SODIUM 153mg; FIBER 16.6g; BETA-CAROTENE 10,174ug; VITAMIN C 71mg; CALCIUM 278mg; IRON 9.3mg; FOLATE 571ug; MAGNESIUM 218mg; ZINC 3.2mg; SELENIUM 7ug

Cuban Black Beans 🌿

INGREDIENTS

1 cup chopped onion

¾ cup chopped green bell pepper

2 cups no-salt-added or low-sodium tomato juice

4¼ cups cooked black beans* or 3 (15-ounce) cans no-salt-added or low-sodium black beans, drained

1½ cups chopped tomatoes, fresh or packaged in BPA-free cartons

1 cup no-salt-added or low-sodium tomato sauce

4 cloves garlic, minced

1 teaspoon cumin

½ teaspoon garlic powder

¼ teaspoon black pepper

1 tablespoon red wine vinegar

¼ cup fresh cilantro

* Use 1½ cups dried beans; see cooking instructions on page 19.

DIRECTIONS

Heat 1 tablespoon water in a large pan and water-sauté onions and peppers until tender. Add all remaining ingredients except vinegar and cilantro. Bring to a boil. Cover, reduce heat, and simmer 20 to 25 minutes or until vegetables are tender. Stir in vinegar and cilantro.

PER SERVING: CALORIES 255; PROTEIN 15g; CARBOHYDRATES 46g; TOTAL FAT 3g; SATURATED FAT 0.5g; SODIUM 82mg; FIBER 14g; BETA-CAROTENE 1,259ug; VITAMIN C 51mg; CALCIUM 73mg; IRON 3.6mg; FOLATE 218ug; MAGNESIUM 114mg; ZINC 1.8mg; SELENIUM 2.8ug

Mushroom and Chickpea Sofrito in Rainbow Chard with Spiced Plum Salad 🌿

>> Executive Chef Martin Oswald

A sofrito is a seasoned, tomato-based sauce used as a foundation in Caribbean, Latin American, and Spanish cooking.

SERVES 6

INGREDIENTS

FOR THE SWISS CHARD:

1 yellow onion, chopped

4 cloves garlic, chopped

1 green pepper, diced

1 red bell pepper, roasted, seeded, and diced

1 teaspoon Spanish paprika

¼ teaspoon saffron threads

Pinch of Mexican chili flakes

½ cup white wine

1 cup diced tomatoes

2 cups cremini mushrooms, roughly chopped and sautéed

2 cups cooked garbanzo beans (chickpeas), roughly chopped

12 blanched Swiss chard leaves, cut into squares

FOR THE PLUM SALAD:

4 plums, or Asian or Bosc pears, sliced

½ cup thinly sliced fennel

2 tablespoons parsley leaves

1 tablespoon aged sherry vinegar or balsamic vinegar

1 tablespoon raw sunflower seeds, crushed

1 tablespoon chives, cut into ½-inch sticks

Pinch of chili flakes

DIRECTIONS

Preheat the oven to 350°F.

Sauté onions and garlic in a hot, dry pan, stirring constantly. Add peppers, paprika, saffron, and chili flakes and toast for 1 minute. Add white wine and tomatoes and reduce slowly for 30 minutes. Remove from heat. Mix in mushrooms and chickpeas.

Place ½ cup mixture on top of each Swiss chard square. Form "raviolis" by folding over the Swiss chard leaves. Place in a casserole dish, cover, and bake for 15 minutes or until heated through.

Combine plum salad ingredients.

Serve topped with plum salad.

PER SERVING: CALORIES 186; PROTEIN 10g; CARBOHYDRATES 33g; TOTAL FAT 1.6g; SATURATED FAT 0.2g; SODIUM 66mg; FIBER 9.4g; BETA-CAROTENE 1,547ug; VITAMIN C 61mg; CALCIUM 94mg; IRON 3.5mg; FOLATE 91ug; MAGNESIUM 84mg; ZINC 1.4mg; SELENIUM 4.5ug

Red Quinoa, Roasted Rainbow Carrots, Brussels Sprouts, Pearl Onions, and Dulse Salad with Pumpkin Seeds and Verjus

>> Chef Jack Hunt

Verjus is the pressed juice of unripened grapes. While acidic, it has a gentler flavor than vinegar. Unlike wine, verjus is not fermented and is not alcoholic. It is available in gourmet food stores or directly from producers. If you are unable to find verjus, substitute 1 cup low-sodium vegetable juice plus 1 tablespoon lemon juice or rice wine vinegar.

SERVES 4

INGREDIENTS:

⅔ cup uncooked red or black quinoa

1 cup pearl onions, peeled (cut larger ones in half)

1 cup diced rainbow carrots (see Note)

½ cup diced celery

1½ cups brussels sprouts, cored and finely shredded in a food processor

2 cloves garlic, minced

1 Serrano or jalapeño chili, minced

1 large pinch dulse flakes

½ cup dried fruit (raisins, currants, chopped unsulfured apricots or figs)

½ cup raw pumpkin seeds

1½ cup verjus

Black pepper to taste

2 tablespoons chopped fresh thyme

2 tablespoons chopped fresh Italian parsley

DIRECTIONS

Wash quinoa thoroughly in cold water in a bowl, then drain through a fine-screen strainer. In a large saucepan, bring quinoa and 2 cups water to a boil. Reduce heat and simmer, uncovered, until grains are translucent and the mixture is the consistency of a thick porridge, about 15 to 20 minutes.

Heat a large sauté pan (cast iron, nonstick, or stainless steel) on high heat. When very hot, reduce heat to medium, add the pearl onions, and sear until golden but not cooked fully. Remove pearl onions and set aside in a small bowl.

Add the carrots, celery, and brussels sprouts and sauté until golden. Add the garlic, chilies, dulse, dried fruit, and pumpkin seeds and sauté lightly for 1 minute. Place pearl onions back into the pan and add the verjus (be careful, there will be a lot of steam coming up from the pan). Scrape any browned bits stuck to the pan with a wooden spoon or high-heat spatula. Season with black pepper, cover, and reduce to medium-low heat. Continue cooking until vegetables are just tender.

Add thyme, parsley, and cooked quinoa and toss together until quinoa has warmed.

NOTE: *Rainbow carrots are red, white, yellow, and purple and are available in gourmet food stores. If you can't find them, substitute regular orange carrots.*

PER SERVING: CALORIES 361; PROTEIN 15g; CARBOHYDRATES 50g; TOTAL FAT 14g; SATURATED FAT 2.5g; SODIUM 56mg; FIBER 6.8g; BETA-CAROTENE 2,914ug; VITAMIN C 47mg; CALCIUM 88mg; IRON 8.2mg; FOLATE 75ug; MAGNESIUM 238mg; ZINC 3.5mg; SELENIUM 2.7ug

Black Bean Spaghetti and Vegetables with Thai Coconut Sauce

» Chef James Rohrbacher

SERVES 6

INGREDIENTS

- 2 cups coconut milk beverage
- 4 (4-inch) stalks lemongrass, broken up into small pieces
- Peel of 1 organic lime, with pith removed
- 1-inch piece ginger, peeled and minced
- ¾ cup unsweetened shredded coconut
- 6 dates, pitted
- ½ tablespoon lime juice
- ⅛ teaspoon cayenne pepper, or more to taste
- 2 tablespoons water or white wine
- 2 cloves garlic
- 3 cups broccoli florets, cut into bite-size pieces
- ½ cup carrots, sliced in ¼-inch pieces
- 8 ounces baby corn ears
- 10 ounces mushrooms, sliced
- 3 cups sliced bok choy
- 1 (7-ounce) package black bean spaghetti
- ¼ cup raw macadamia nuts, raw cashews, or raw Spanish peanuts, lightly toasted

DIRECTIONS

Place coconut milk beverage, lemongrass, lime peel, and ginger in a saucepan. Bring to a boil, remove from heat, cover and let steep for 30 minutes. Mash lemongrass, lime peel, and ginger into mixture with a wooden spoon. Pour through a fine-mesh strainer to remove fibers. Add coconut milk to a high-powered blender along with shredded coconut, dates, lime juice, and cayenne pepper. Blend until smooth and creamy.

In a large wok or skillet, heat water or white wine, add garlic, broccoli, carrots, and baby corn, and stir-fry for 2 minutes, adding more water as needed. Add mushrooms and bok choy and continue to cook until vegetables start to soften, about 4 minutes. Add coconut sauce, cover, and cook for 2 to 3 minutes until vegetables are crisp-tender.

Meanwhile, cook spaghetti according to package directions.

Serve pasta topped with vegetables and sauce. Sprinkle with lightly toasted nuts.

PER SERVING: CALORIES 401; PROTEIN 16g; CARBOHYDRATES 65g; TOTAL FAT 11.4g; SATURATED FAT 4.2g; SODIUM 92mg; FIBER 5.5g; BETA-CAROTENE 1,301ug; VITAMIN C 49mg; CALCIUM 102mg; IRON 4.4mg; FOLATE 87ug; MAGNESIUM 138mg; ZINC 2.6mg; SELENIUM 39.6ug

Mediterranean Bean and Kale Sauté

SERVES 4

INGREDIENTS

½ cup unsulfured, no-salt, no-oil-added dried tomatoes, soaked for 30 minutes in hot water to cover

2 bunches kale, tough stems and center ribs removed, chopped

1 medium onion, finely chopped

1 cup shiitake mushrooms, coarsely chopped

3 cloves garlic, pressed

1 cup cooked* or canned, no-salt-added or low-sodium beans, any type

1½ tablespoons sherry vinegar

1 tablespoon Dijon mustard

Red pepper flakes to taste

½ cup no-salt-added or low-sodium pasta sauce

¼ cup Nutritarian "Parmesan" (see box on page 234)

* Use ⅓ cup dried beans; see cooking instructions on page 19.

DIRECTIONS

Drain dried tomatoes, reserving soaking water. Chop.

Heat tomato-soaking water in a large skillet and sauté the kale, tomatoes, onion, mushrooms, and garlic over medium heat for 5 minutes, adding additional water as needed. Cover and steam for 10 minutes.

Add the beans, vinegar, mustard, and red pepper flakes and cook for 3 more minutes or until mushrooms are tender and liquid cooks out.

Toss with pasta sauce. Serve topped with "Parmesan" cheese.

PER SERVING: CALORIES 221; PROTEIN 10g; CARBOHYDRATES 32g; TOTAL FAT 7.3g; SATURATED FAT 0.7g; SODIUM 304mg; FIBER 7g; BETA-CAROTENE 6,939ug; VITAMIN C 96mg; CALCIUM 173mg; IRON 3.9mg; FOLATE 85ug; MAGNESIUM 95mg; ZINC 1.9mg; SELENIUM 8.7ug

Remember the most powerful, longevity-promoting foods:

G-BOMBS

Greens • Beans • Onions • Mushrooms • Berries • Seeds

FUHRMAN FAST FOOD

*Recipes recommended for aggressive weight-loss
and diabetic diets and for people
with metabolic syndrome are marked with 🌿.*

FUHRMAN FAST FOOD

Fast food doesn't have to be unhealthy. In this chapter, I have included a variety of delicious recipes for burgers, pizza, and sandwiches. To make your own quick and easy wraps, mix and match some of these options:

GUIDE TO CONSTRUCTING HEALTHY WRAPS

HEALTHY "WRAP" MATERIAL	FILLING	SPREAD/ TOPPING	ADD-ONS
100% whole-grain flour tortilla	avocado	Russian Fig Dressing (page 91) or other healthy dips and dressings (page 79)	raw chopped nuts
100% whole-grain pita	tomato		raw seeds
Boston lettuce leaves	chopped onion		fresh basil, cilantro, or mint
collard green leaves	shredded lettuce		dried oregano
	watercress/ arugula	hummus	unsulfured, dried tomatoes, soaked
	spinach	black beans pureed with tomato	banana slices/ ripe plantain
	chopped cucumber	mashed beans	apple slices
	grated carrot or beet	raw cashew or almond butter	dried fruit (presoaked)
	red/green bell pepper or jalapeño slices	tahini	
	grilled portobello mushrooms		

Sunny Bean Burgers 🌿

SERVES 2

INGREDIENTS

Small amount of olive oil

¼ cup raw sunflower seeds

2 cups cooked kidney or pinto beans or canned no-salt-added or low-sodium kidney beans, drained

½ cup minced onion

2 tablespoons low-sodium ketchup

1 tablespoon wheat germ or old-fashioned rolled oats

½ teaspoon chili powder

DIRECTIONS

Preheat the oven to 350°F. Lightly oil a baking sheet with a little olive oil on a paper towel.

Chop the sunflower seeds in a food processor or with a hand chopper. Mash the beans in the food processor or with a potato masher and mix with the sunflower seeds. Mix in the remaining ingredients and form into six patties.

Place the patties on the baking sheet and bake for 25 minutes. Remove from the oven and let cool slightly, until you can pick up each patty and compress it firmly in your hands to re-form the burger. Return the patties to the baking sheet, bottom side up, and bake for another 10 minutes.

NOTE: If desired, these may be cooked on a grill.

PER SERVING: CALORIES 123; PROTEIN 6g; CARBOHYDRATES 18g; TOTAL FAT 3.6g; SATURATED FAT 0.4g; SODIUM 5mg; FIBER 5.4g; BETA-CAROTENE 61ug; VITAMIN C 3mg; CALCIUM 24mg; IRON 2.2mg; FOLATE 94ug; MAGNESIUM 39mg; ZINC 1mg; SELENIUM 1.1ug

Better Burgers 🌿

INGREDIENTS

- 1½ cups old-fashioned rolled oats
- 1 cup ground walnuts
- 1 cup water
- ¼ cup tomato paste
- No-salt seasoning blend, adjusted to taste, or ¼ cup Dr. Fuhrman's MatoZest
- 1 cup diced onion
- 3 cloves garlic, minced
- 6 cups finely minced mushrooms
- 2 teaspoons dried basil
- ½ teaspoon dried oregano
- 2 tablespoons minced fresh parsley
- Freshly ground pepper to taste
- ⅔ cup frozen chopped spinach, thawed

DIRECTIONS

Preheat the oven to 350°F.

Combine rolled oats and ground walnuts in a bowl. Set aside.

In a small saucepan, whisk together water, tomato paste, and MatoZest or other no-salt seasoning blend. Heat over medium-high heat until boiling. Pour over rolled oats and walnuts. Stir well and set aside.

Heat 2 tablespoons water in a sauté pan and add onion and garlic. Sauté until onion is translucent. Add mushrooms, basil, oregano, parsley, black pepper, and additional water, if needed to prevent sticking. Cover and cook for 5 minutes, or until mushrooms are tender.

In a large bowl, combine sautéed onions and mushrooms, rolled oat/walnut mixture, and spinach. Stir well to combine. With wet hands, shape ⅓ cup of mixture into a well-formed burger. Place on a lightly oiled baking sheet and repeat with remaining mixture. Bake for 15 minutes. Turn burgers to bake the other side for another 15 minutes.

Remove from the oven and cool slightly. Serve on small, whole-grain hamburger buns or whole-grain pita bread halves. Top with thinly sliced, raw red onion and no-salt or low-sodium ketchup.

Makes 8 burgers.

NOTE: If desired, 8 ounces of ground turkey breast may be mixed in before forming the patties.

PER SERVING: CALORIES 199; PROTEIN 9g; CARBOHYDRATES 21g; TOTAL FAT 11.1g; SATURATED FAT 1.1g; SODIUM 101mg; FIBER 4.4g; BETA-CAROTENE 1,642ug; VITAMIN C 12mg; CALCIUM 50mg; IRON 2.5mg; FOLATE 55ug; MAGNESIUM 86mg; ZINC 1.5mg; SELENIUM 14.1ug

Sweet Potato Black Bean Burgers 🌿

SERVES 6

INGREDIENTS

⅓ cup raw cashews

⅓ cup raw pecans

1½ cups cooked black beans* or 1 (15-ounce) can no-salt-added or low-sodium black beans, drained

¾ cup baked sweet potato, mashed

½ cup diced red onion

½ jalapeño pepper, deseeded and diced

3 tablespoons chopped cilantro

1 teaspoon garlic powder

½ teaspoon black pepper

1 tablespoon cider vinegar

2 tablespoons fresh lime juice

3 tablespoons nutritional yeast

Small amount of olive oil or olive oil cooking spray

*Use ½ cup dried beans; see cooking instructions on page 19.

DIRECTIONS

Preheat the oven to 350°F.

Place nuts in a food processor and grind to a fine powder. Add remaining ingredients, except for olive oil, and pulse to combine.

Form mixture into 6 burgers. Place on a baking pan that has been rubbed lightly with olive oil or sprayed with cooking spray. Bake for 30 minutes until lightly browned.

Serve with avocado, tomato, and red onion slices.

PER SERVING: CALORIES 163; PROTEIN 8g; CARBOHYDRATES 22g; TOTAL FAT 5.6g; SATURATED FAT 1.1g; SODIUM 18mg; FIBER 6.4g; BETA-CAROTENE 2,967ug; VITAMIN C 9mg; CALCIUM 40mg; IRON 2.5mg; FOLATE 234ug; MAGNESIUM 77mg; ZINC 1.5mg; SELENIUM 2.1ug

Kyoto Mushroom Burgers 🌿

SERVES 6-8

INGREDIENTS

- ½ cup chopped red onion
- 2 cups chopped portobello mushrooms
- ½ cup chopped carrots
- ½ cup peeled and chopped zucchini
- 2 cloves garlic, minced
- 1 teaspoon white miso
- 1 cup cooked brown rice
- ½ cup raw sunflower seeds, ground
- 2 tablespoons chopped fresh parsley
- 2 tablespoons chopped fresh basil
- 1 cup whole-wheat bread crumbs
- Olive oil (small amount)

DIRECTIONS

Preheat the oven to 300°F.

Heat ⅛ cup water in a large frying pan over medium heat. Water-sauté onions, mushrooms, carrots, zucchini, and garlic about 10 minutes or until vegetables are tender, adding more water if needed to prevent sticking. Add miso and blend well.

In a food processor, add sautéed vegetables, cooked rice, sunflower seeds, parsley, and basil and pulse several times until well mixed.

Add bread crumbs and pulse again until all the ingredients hold together.

Rub a baking pan with a small amount of olive oil. Shape mixture into 3½ by ½ inch burgers and bake for 10 minutes on each side, until firm.

Makes 6–8 burgers.

PER SERVING: CALORIES 147; PROTEIN 6g; CARBOHYDRATES 18g; TOTAL FAT 6.7g; SATURATED FAT 0.8g; SODIUM 82mg; FIBER 3.5g; BETA-CAROTENE 948ug; VITAMIN C 6mg; CALCIUM 40mg; IRON 1.6mg; FOLATE 48ug; MAGNESIUM 72mg; ZINC 1.2mg; SELENIUM 16.9ug

Bean Enchiladas 🌱

INGREDIENTS

1 medium green bell pepper, seeded and chopped

½ cup sliced onion

8 ounces no-salt-added or low-sodium tomato sauce, divided

2 cups cooked pinto or black beans* or canned no-salt-added or low-sodium beans, drained

1 cup frozen corn kernels

1 tablespoon chili powder

1 teaspoon ground cumin

1 teaspoon onion powder

1 tablespoon chopped fresh cilantro

⅛ teaspoon cayenne pepper, or to taste

6 corn tortillas

* Use ⅔ cup dried beans; see cooking instructions on page 19.

DIRECTIONS

Preheat the oven to 375°F (optional).

Sauté the green pepper and onion in 2 tablespoons of the tomato sauce until tender. Stir in the remaining tomato sauce, beans, corn, chili powder, cumin, onion powder, cilantro, and cayenne (if using). Simmer for 5 minutes. Spoon about ¼ cup of the bean mixture on each tortilla and roll up. Serve as is or bake for 15 minutes.

PER SERVING: CALORIES 187; PROTEIN 8g; CARBOHYDRATES 37g; TOTAL FAT 1.7g; SATURATED FAT 0.3g; SODIUM 33mg; FIBER 9g; BETA-CAROTENE 351ug; VITAMIN C 25mg; CALCIUM 57mg; IRON 2.2mg; FOLATE 107ug; MAGNESIUM 77mg; ZINC 1.3mg; SELENIUM 2.9ug

Veg-Head Bean Burrito 🌿

SERVES 6

INGREDIENTS

1 head broccoli florets, chopped

½ head cauliflower florets, chopped

2 carrots, chopped

2 medium red bell peppers, seeded and chopped

1 medium zucchini, chopped

1 medium onion, chopped

4 cloves garlic, chopped

½ teaspoon chili powder

½ teaspoon ground cumin

1 teaspoon dried oregano

½ cup raw cashews

½ cup raw almonds

½ cup unsweetened soy, hemp, or almond milk

1½ cups cooked pinto beans or 1 (15-ounce) can no-salt-added or low-sodium pinto beans, drained

6 whole-wheat tortillas or large romaine lettuce leaves

Salsa (page 96)

DIRECTIONS

Place 2 tablespoons water, the broccoli, cauliflower, carrots, bell peppers, zucchini, onion, garlic, chili powder, cumin, and oregano in a large covered pot. Sauté for 15 minutes or until tender, adding more water if needed. In the meantime, place nuts and milk in a food processor or high-powered blender and blend until smooth. Add the cashew mixture and beans to the vegetables and mix thoroughly. Spread the mixture on the tortillas or lettuce leaves and roll up to form burritos. Serve with salsa.

PER SERVING: CALORIES 524; PROTEIN 20g; CARBOHYDRATES 78g; TOTAL FAT 17.2g; SATURATED FAT 3.6g; SODIUM 447mg; FIBER 14.7g; BETA-CAROTENE 3,666ug; VITAMIN C 167mg; CALCIUM 154mg; IRON 6.2mg; FOLATE 385ug; MAGNESIUM 151mg; ZINC 3.2mg; SELENIUM 25.8ug

Portobello Veggie Fajitas 🌱

SERVES 4

INGREDIENTS

4 portobello mushroom caps, cut into strips

2 green bell peppers, cut into strips

2 small yellow squash, cut into strips

1 medium white onion, chopped

½ Serrano chili, seeded, minced

1 garlic clove, chopped

1 tablespoon chili powder, or to taste

1 cup cooked beans* (any type) or canned low-sodium or no-salt-added beans, drained

3 tablespoons chopped fresh cilantro

4 large whole-grain tortillas

Salsa (page 96)

1 avocado, peeled and sliced

* Use ⅓ cup dried beans; see cooking instructions on page 19.

DIRECTIONS

Combine mushrooms, green peppers, squash, onion, Serrano chili, garlic, and chili powder. Heat 2 tablespoons water in a skillet and water-sauté veggies until tender, about 5 minutes, adding extra water if needed to prevent sticking. Add beans and cook until heated through. Stir in cilantro.

Serve on warmed tortillas topped with salsa and sliced avocado.

PER SERVING: CALORIES 411; PROTEIN 14g; CARBOHYDRATES 64g; TOTAL FAT 12.4g; SATURATED FAT 2.3g; SODIUM 375mg; FIBER 11.1g; BETA-CAROTENE 514ug; VITAMIN C 65mg; CALCIUM 102mg; IRON 5.1mg; FOLATE 196ug; MAGNESIUM 83mg; ZINC 1.9mg; SELENIUM 19.8ug

Roasted Vegetable Pizza

SERVES 2

INGREDIENTS

- 2 cups broccoli florets
- 1 large red bell pepper, cut into 1-inch slices
- 1 large portobello mushroom, cut into ½-inch slices
- 1 teaspoon garlic powder
- 1 tablespoon balsamic vinegar
- ½ teaspoon dried oregano
- 5 ounces organic baby spinach
- ½ cup no-salt-added or low-sodium pasta sauce
- 2 whole-grain tortillas or whole-wheat pita bread
- 2 tablespoons mozzarella-type, nondairy cheese, shredded

DIRECTIONS

Preheat the oven to 350°F.

Toss broccoli, bell peppers, and mushrooms with garlic powder, balsamic vinegar, and oregano. Roast seasoned vegetables on a cookie sheet for 20 minutes, turning occasionally and mounding to keep from drying out.

Steam spinach until just wilted.

Spread a layer of pasta sauce on tortilla or on top of pita bread, sprinkle lightly with nondairy cheese, and distribute roasted vegetables and spinach on top.

Bake for approximately 7 minutes or until cheese is melted.

PER SERVING: CALORIES 388; PROTEIN 14g; CARBOHYDRATES 64g; TOTAL FAT 9.8g; SATURATED FAT 2g; SODIUM 498mg; FIBER 7.5g; BETA-CAROTENE 5,376ug; VITAMIN C 170mg; CALCIUM 200mg; IRON 6mg; FOLATE 318ug; MAGNESIUM 222mg; ZINC 1.8mg; SELENIUM 25.6ug

Italian Stuffer

>> Chef Christine Waltermyer

SERVES 2

INGREDIENTS

. . . .

¼ cup unsulfured, unsalted, dried tomatoes

2 cups shredded lettuce

¼ cup chopped parsley

½ cup finely ground walnuts

1 teaspoon Italian seasoning

1½ tablespoons tomato paste

Pinch of garlic powder

Thinly sliced red onion

2 (100% whole-grain) pitas or tortillas

DIRECTIONS

. . . .

Soak dried tomatoes, for 30 minutes, in just enough water to cover. Drain, reserving soaking water, and chop.

In a bowl, mix soaked tomatoes and soaking water with lettuce, parsley, walnuts, seasoning, tomato paste, and garlic powder. Along with sliced onion, stuff into whole-grain pitas or place on tortillas and roll up.

NOTE: If desired, 1–2 ounces sliced or chopped oven-baked chicken or turkey breast may be added to each wrap.

. . . .

PER SERVING: CALORIES 413; PROTEIN 14g; CARBOHYDRATES 50g; TOTAL FAT 21.2g; SATURATED FAT 2.1g; SODIUM 370mg; FIBER 10g; BETA-CAROTENE 2,679ug; VITAMIN C 31mg; CALCIUM 84mg; IRON 5mg; FOLATE 148ug; MAGNESIUM 122mg; ZINC 2.2mg; SELENIUM 31ug

Popeye Pitas with Mediterranean Tomato Spread 🌿

SERVES 4

INGREDIENTS

FOR THE SPREAD:

1 cup cooked* or canned great northern beans, low-sodium or no-salt-added, drained

¼ cup pine nuts (see Note)

2 tablespoons unsulfured, unsalted, dried tomatoes, minced

1 clove garlic

No-salt seasoning blend, adjusted to taste, or 1 teaspoon Dr. Fuhrman's MatoZest

1 teaspoon balsamic vinegar

½ teaspoon minced fresh rosemary, if desired

* Use ⅓ cup dried beans; see cooking instructions on page 19.

FOR THE SANDWICH:

4 whole-wheat pitas

1 tomato, sliced

½ cup thinly sliced red onion

2 cups finely chopped arugula

2 cups finely chopped spinach

1 avocado, sliced

DIRECTIONS

Combine spread ingredients in a high-powdered blender or food processor until smooth.

Toast pitas, slice open a top slit, and spread apart. Stuff with sandwich ingredients and spread.

NOTE: Use Mediterranean pine nuts if available. Chopped almonds may be substituted. See box on page 90.

PER SERVING: CALORIES 387; PROTEIN 15g; CARBOHYDRATES 57g; TOTAL FAT 14.5g; SATURATED FAT 1.7g; SODIUM 365mg; FIBER 12.1g; BETA-CAROTENE 1,262ug; VITAMIN C 16mg; CALCIUM 99mg; IRON 5.3mg; FOLATE 147ug; MAGNESIUM 132mg; ZINC 2.7mg; SELENIUM 29.4ug

Portobello Red Pepper Sandwich ✎

SERVES 4

INGREDIENTS

FOR THE SANDWICH:

4 large portobello mushrooms, stems removed

½ large red onion, thinly sliced

4 whole-grain pitas

2 cups large arugula leaves

2 medium roasted red bell peppers, drained, seeded, and cut into ½-inch-thick slices

FOR THE SPREAD:

½ cup tahini (pureed sesame seeds) or ⅔ cup unhulled sesame seeds

½ cup water

1 tablespoon fresh lemon juice

No-salt seasoning blend, adjusted to taste, or 1 tablespoon Dr. Fuhrman's VegiZest

1 teaspoon Bragg Liquid Aminos or low-sodium soy sauce

2 pitted dates, chopped

1 small clove garlic, chopped

DIRECTIONS

Preheat the oven to 375°F. Arrange mushrooms and onions on a baking sheet and roast until tender, about 15 to 20 minutes.

Meanwhile, make tahini spread by blending all ingredients together until creamy in a food processor or high-powered blender. (If using whole sesame seeds, first blend sesame seeds with ¼ cup water until creamy and then add the other ¼ cup water and remaining ingredients.)

When mushrooms/onions are done, split pitas in half horizontally and warm slightly. Spread generous amount of tahini on top half of split pita. Place ½ cup arugula on bottom half and then 1 mushroom cap (patted dry with paper towels to absorb liquid), sliced onion, and roasted red pepper.

PER SERVING: CALORIES 392; PROTEIN 14g; CARBOHYDRATES 52g; TOTAL FAT 18g; SATURATED FAT 2.5g; SODIUM 442mg; FIBER 7.7g; BETA-CAROTENE 443ug; VITAMIN C 7mg; CALCIUM 80mg; IRON 4mg; FOLATE 78ug; MAGNESIUM 87mg; ZINC 2.8mg; SELENIUM 35.2ug

Vegetable Garbanzo Wraps 🌿

INGREDIENTS

1½ cups cooked garbanzo beans* (chickpeas) or 1 (15-ounce) can low-sodium or no-salt-added garbanzo beans, drained

1 large tomato, chopped

1 avocado, chopped

1 cucumber, chopped

4 leaves romaine lettuce, shredded

2 tablespoons white balsamic vinegar or Dr. Fuhrman's Riesling Reserve Vinegar

4 whole-grain tortillas

½ tablespoon tahini (pureed sesame seeds)

* Use ½ cup dried beans; see cooking instructions on page 19.

DIRECTIONS

Mash garbanzo beans. Toss with tomato, avocado, cucumber, lettuce, and vinegar.

Warm a whole-grain tortilla, spread a thin coating of tahini on it, top with the vegetable/bean mixture, and roll up.

PER SERVING: CALORIES 318; PROTEIN 12g; CARBOHYDRATES 45g; TOTAL FAT 11.8g; SATURATED FAT 1.8g; SODIUM 222mg; FIBER 10.8g; BETA-CAROTENE 2,223ug; VITAMIN C 26mg; CALCIUM 121mg; IRON 4.1mg; FOLATE 267ug; MAGNESIUM 74mg; ZINC 1.8mg; SELENIUM 10.8ug

Black Bean Lettuce Bundles 🌿

SERVES 4

INGREDIENTS

2 cups cooked* or canned no-salt-added or low-sodium black beans, drained

½ large ripe avocado, peeled, pitted, and mashed

½ medium green bell pepper, seeded and chopped

3 green onions, chopped

⅓ cup chopped fresh cilantro

⅓ cup mild, no-salt-added or low-sodium salsa

2 tablespoons fresh lime juice

1 clove garlic, minced

1 teaspoon ground cumin

8 large romaine lettuce leaves

* Use ⅔ cup dried beans; see cooking instructions on page 19.

DIRECTIONS

In a bowl, mash the beans and avocado together with a fork until well blended and only slightly chunky. Add all the remaining ingredients, except the lettuce, and mix.

Place approximately ¼ cup of the mixture in the center of each lettuce leaf and roll up like a burrito.

PER SERVING: CALORIES 171; PROTEIN 10g; CARBOHYDRATES 27g; TOTAL FAT 4.1g; SATURATED FAT 0.6g; SODIUM 13mg; FIBER 11g; BETA-CAROTENE 2,470ug; VITAMIN C 26mg; CALCIUM 63mg; IRON 2.8mg; FOLATE 231ug; MAGNESIUM 80mg; ZINC 1.3mg; SELENIUM 1.6ug

Collard Dijon Wraps 🌿

SERVES 2

INGREDIENTS

- 4 prunes (reduce to 2 prunes for diabetic and weight-loss diets)
- 2 teaspoons Dijon mustard
- 2 teaspoons red wine vinegar
- 2 tablespoons shredded carrots
- 2 tablespoons shredded cucumber
- ¼ cup chopped red onion
- ¼ cup chopped bell pepper, green or red
- 2 large collard leaves, thick stems removed
- 2 medium romaine leaves
- 4 tomato slices
- ½ avocado, cut into 4 slices

DIRECTIONS

Soak prunes for 30 minutes in enough water to cover. Drain and chop. Combine the Dijon mustard, prunes, and red wine vinegar in a medium bowl and mash with a fork. Stir in carrots, cucumber, red onion, and pepper.

Lay out a large collard leaf and place a romaine leaf on top of it. Top with half of the mustard/vegetable mixture and 2 slices of tomato and avocado. Roll like a burrito.

PER SERVING: CALORIES 150; PROTEIN 4g; CARBOHYDRATES 18g; TOTAL FAT 8g; SATURATED FAT 1.5g; SODIUM 136mg; FIBER 7.3g; BETA-CAROTENE 2,816ug; VITAMIN C 56mg; CALCIUM 58mg; IRON 0.8mg; FOLATE 113ug; MAGNESIUM 36mg; ZINC 0.6mg; SELENIUM 0.5ug

Korean Vegetable and Mushroom Lettuce Wraps 🌿

The vegetables in these wraps can be stir-fried for a quick meal or pickled for an authentic Korean flavor. Since the vegetables need two days to "pickle," plan ahead and do some extra vegetables to keep on hand for other uses. They will keep in the refrigerator for three to four weeks.

SERVES 4

INGREDIENTS

FOR THE VEGETABLES:

1 medium onion, sliced

4 cups small broccoli florets

2 medium carrots, cut diagonally into ⅓-inch pieces

4 medium red bell peppers, seeded and cut into 1-inch squares

2 cups bok choy, cut in bite-size pieces

3 cups fresh mushrooms (shiitake, porcini, and/or cremini), stems removed

1 pound fresh spinach

FOR THE DRESSING:

⅓ cup raw almond butter

¼ cup unsweetened soy, almond, or hemp milk

¼ cup water

3 tablespoons unhulled sesame seeds

2 dates, pitted

2 cloves garlic, chopped

½-inch piece fresh ginger, peeled and chopped

Pinch of hot pepper flakes, or more to taste

FOR SERVING:

Romaine, Boston or other lettuce leaves, large enough to use as a wrap

DIRECTIONS

For pickled vegetables, see recipe for Nutritarian Pickling Juice on page 110. Allow 2 days for vegetables to pickle.

If you are not pickling your vegetables, heat 2 tablespoons water in a large sauté pan and water-sauté the onion, broccoli, carrots, and bell peppers for 5 minutes, adding more water as necessary to keep vegetables from scorching. Add the bok choy and mushrooms, cover, and simmer until vegetables are just tender. Remove the cover and cook off most of the water. Add the spinach and toss until wilted.

Blend all dressing ingredients together in a high-powered blender until creamy. Add more water as necessary to adjust consistency.

To serve, spoon filling onto a lettuce leaf, add a bit of dressing, and roll up.

PER SERVING: CALORIES 339; PROTEIN 16g; CARBOHYDRATES 39g; TOTAL FAT 17.7g; SATURATED FAT 1.9g; SODIUM 175mg; FIBER 13.2g; BETA-CAROTENE 13,175ug; VITAMIN C 290mg; CALCIUM 350mg; IRON 7.5mg; FOLATE 465ug; MAGNESIUM 243mg; ZINC 3.2mg; SELENIUM 12.3ug

Spiced Sweet Potato Cornbread

» Talia Fuhrman

SERVES 10

INGREDIENTS

1 cup cornmeal

1 cup oat flour

1 tablespoon baking powder

12 Medjool dates or 24 regular dates, pitted

1 cup coconut milk beverage

¼ cup unsweetened shredded coconut

1 cup baked and peeled sweet potato

2 tablespoons ground flax seeds

1 teaspoon ground cinnamon

½ teaspoon ground nutmeg

¼ teaspoon ground cloves

1 cup frozen corn kernels

DIRECTIONS

Preheat the oven to 375°F.

Combine cornmeal, oat flour, and baking powder in a large bowl. Stir well and set the bowl aside.

In a high-powered blender, combine dates, coconut milk beverage, coconut, sweet potato, ground flax seeds, and spices. Combine with the dry ingredients, stirring just until well combined. Add in frozen corn kernels.

Pour the batter into a nonstick square baking dish, cast iron skillet, or even bake as individual muffins. Bake for 30 minutes or until the top has a golden tinge. Cool for 10 to 15 minutes before serving.

PER SERVING: CALORIES 229; PROTEIN 5g; CARBOHYDRATES 49g; TOTAL FAT 3.1g; SATURATED FAT 0.9g; SODIUM 25mg; FIBER 5.5g; BETA-CAROTENE 2,438ug; VITAMIN C 5mg; CALCIUM 114mg; IRON 2.1mg; FOLATE 47ug; MAGNESIUM 42mg; ZINC 0.6mg; SELENIUM 3.5ug

NONVEGAN DISHES

Recipes recommended for aggressive weight-loss and diabetic diets and for people with metabolic syndrome are marked with 🌿.

NONVEGAN DISHES

The use of animal products in a nutritarian diet is optional. One can be vegan, near-vegan, or flexitarian, using animal products semi-regularly but in very small amounts, and overall, be eating healthfully. If you want to use animal products in your diet, don't eat a large portion at any meal. Instead use them in small amounts more as a condiment or flavoring.

I recommend that you restrict animal-source products (meat, dairy, and eggs) to two or fewer servings per week and only one or two ounces at a time. The recipes that follow contain approximately 2 ounces of animal product per serving.

A review of the scientific literature supports the conclusion that, if animal products are consumed, they should constitute no more than 10 percent of total caloric intake. As these foods increase in the diet, the modern diseases that kill over 80 percent of Americans (heart disease, stroke, cancer, and diabetes) occur in greater and greater likelihood.

Foods of animal origin are high in calories and very low in nutrients per calorie compared to vegetables. The higher your animal product consumption, the lower your nutrient intake. Diets rich in animal protein are also associated with high blood levels of the hormone IGF-1, which is a known risk factor for several types of cancer. I discuss this in detail in my book *Super Immunity.*

If you do choose to include a small amount of meat in your diet, select certified organic products. You can be sure that the feed is grown without chemical pesticides and the animal is not treated with antibiotics or hormones. Organic farms are monitored and the producers are held responsible for their practices. "Natural" meats may follow some or all of the organic practices but they do not have to. "Natural" and "grass-fed" are voluntary terms and are not monitored. They can refer to a wide range of attributes.

Garden Eggs and Tofu with Salsa

SERVES 3

INGREDIENTS

½ medium onion, diced

1 medium zucchini, grated

1 carrot, grated

2 cups chopped Swiss chard or organic spinach

½ medium tomato, diced

2 cloves garlic, pressed

2 teaspoons herbes de Provence

1 cup firm tofu

⅛ teaspoon curry powder, or more to taste

3 eggs, beaten

¼ cup no-salt-added or low-sodium salsa

1 ounce nondairy, mozzarella-type cheese, grated

DIRECTIONS

In a large sauté pan, heat ⅛ cup water and water-sauté the onion, zucchini, carrot, and Swiss chard for about 2 minutes. Add the tomato, garlic, and herbs. Cook, stirring, for about 2 minutes, until the vegetables begin to soften.

Squeeze water out of tofu and crumble.

Scatter the tofu over the vegetables and sprinkle with curry powder.

Mix with vegetables and cook over high heat until water is cooked away.

Reduce the heat to low and stir in the eggs, mixing well so the vegetables and tofu bind with the eggs. Continue stirring until the eggs are cooked.

Top with salsa and grated cheese.

PER SERVING: CALORIES 261; PROTEIN 24g; CARBOHYDRATES 17g; TOTAL FAT 13.4g; SATURATED FAT 2.8g; CHOLESTEROL 211mg; SODIUM 291mg; FIBER 4.8g; BETA-CAROTENE 2,776ug; VITAMIN C 26mg; CALCIUM 670mg; IRON 4.7mg; FOLATE 93ug; MAGNESIUM 120mg; ZINC 2.6mg; SELENIUM 33.2ug

Scrambled Veggies and Eggs

SERVES 2

INGREDIENTS

- 2 eggs
- 2 tablespoons unsweetened soy, hemp, or almond milk
- ½ medium bell pepper, diced
- 2 green onions, chopped
- ½ cup diced fresh tomatoes
- 1 cup diced fresh mushrooms
- No-salt seasoning blend, adjusted to taste, or 1 tablespoon Dr. Fuhrman's MatoZest
- 4 ounces spinach, coarsely chopped, or baby spinach
- Freshly ground black pepper to taste

DIRECTIONS

Beat eggs with soy milk.

Heat ⅛ cup water in a sauté pan and add the peppers, onions, tomatoes, mushrooms, and MatoZest or other no-salt seasoning blend. Sauté until vegetables are tender and most of the water is cooked out. Add spinach to wilt.

Add egg mixture and scramble until cooked through. Season with black pepper.

PER SERVING: CALORIES 131; PROTEIN 13g; CARBOHYDRATES 11g; TOTAL FAT 5.8g; SATURATED FAT 1.7g; CHOLESTEROL 211mg; SODIUM 151mg; FIBER 3.3g; BETA-CAROTENE 4,203ug; VITAMIN C 52mg; CALCIUM 108mg; IRON 3.7mg; FOLATE 163ug; MAGNESIUM 70mg; ZINC 1.3mg; SELENIUM 21.7ug

Mediterranean Fish Stew 🌿

SERVES 4

INGREDIENTS

2 red bell peppers, sliced

2 medium onions, sliced

1 medium eggplant, cut into 1-inch pieces

2 medium zucchini, cut into 1-inch pieces

1 cup sliced mushrooms

6 medium tomatoes, chopped

2 cloves garlic, finely chopped

1 teaspoon herbes de Provence

¼ teaspoon black pepper

½ pound firm fish fillets (such as halibut, bass, salmon), cut into 1-inch pieces

2 tablespoons fresh chopped parsley

1 tablespoon fresh lemon juice

DIRECTIONS

Heat ⅛ cup water in a large pan. Add the bell peppers and onions and cook for 3 minutes. Add the eggplant, zucchini, and mushrooms and continue cooking for another 6 to 8 minutes or until tender, adding more water if necessary to keep from sticking.

Add the tomatoes, garlic, herbes de Provence, and black pepper and simmer on low heat for 4 minutes.

Add the fish to the stew and mix in gently. Cover and simmer on low heat for 8 to 10 minutes, stirring occasionally.

Before serving, stir in parsley and lemon juice.

PER SERVING: CALORIES 192; PROTEIN 23g; CARBOHYDRATES 29g; TOTAL FAT 2.5g; SATURATED FAT 0.4g; CHOLESTEROL 18.1mg; SODIUM 60mg; FIBER 10.7g; BETA-CAROTENE 2,045ug; VITAMIN C 129mg; CALCIUM 102mg; IRON 3mg; FOLATE 139ug; MAGNESIUM 121mg; ZINC 1.5mg; SELENIUM 24.1ug

Salmon and Vegetables in a Packet 🌿

SERVES 4

INGREDIENTS

8 ounces salmon fillets or steaks, divided into 4 pieces

Freshly ground pepper

1 teaspoon freshly grated ginger root

Juice of 1 lemon

3 ripe tomatoes, chopped

2 medium zucchini, chopped

2 cups sliced mushrooms

2 medium red onions, thinly sliced

2 cloves garlic, minced or pressed

4 sheets aluminum foil, 12 x 24 inches

Small amount of olive oil or olive oil cooking spray

4 cups coarsely chopped mustard greens or Swiss chard

DIRECTIONS

Preheat the oven to 450°F.

Place the salmon pieces in a glass baking dish and add pepper, grated ginger, and lemon juice.

In a large bowl, mix tomatoes, zucchini, mushrooms, red onion, and garlic.

Fold each piece of foil over to make a square of double thickness. Brush the center portion of each square with a small amount of olive oil.

On each square, place 1 cup chopped mustard greens, 1 salmon fillet and one-quarter of the tomato/vegetable mixture.

Fold the foil into airtight packets. Bake for 20 minutes. Open packet and check that fish is cooked, being careful to avoid steam that is released.

To serve, open the foil and transfer contents to a plate or bowl.

PER SERVING: CALORIES 226; PROTEIN 30g; CARBOHYDRATES 12g; TOTAL FAT 7.2g; SATURATED FAT 1.5g; CHOLESTEROL 51mg; SODIUM 78mg; FIBER 4.1g; BETA-CAROTENE 3,864ug; VITAMIN C 65mg; CALCIUM 122mg; IRON 2.1mg; FOLATE 153ug; MAGNESIUM 76mg; ZINC 1.1mg; SELENIUM 46.7ug

Creole Chicken and Spinach 🌿

SERVES 4

INGREDIENTS

8 ounces boneless, naturally raised, organic chicken breasts, thinly sliced, crosswise

1 cup chopped celery

1½ cups chopped fresh tomatoes or canned diced tomatoes, no-salt-added or low-sodium

10 ounces frozen spinach

1 large green pepper, chopped

½ cup chopped onion

4 cloves garlic, minced

¾ cup no-salt-added or low-sodium vegetable broth

2 tablespoons tomato paste

1 tablespoon chopped fresh basil or 1 teaspoon dried

2 teaspoons chili powder, or more to taste

1 tablespoon chopped fresh parsley or 1 teaspoon dried

¼ teaspoon dried crushed red pepper, or more to taste

2 cups cooked brown rice and/or wild rice

DIRECTIONS

Cook chicken strips in a lightly oiled skillet, turning occasionally, for 3 to 5 minutes until no longer pink.

Add remaining ingredients, except for rice, bring to a boil, and reduce heat to medium. Simmer covered for 10 minutes or until vegetables are tender.

Serve over rice.

PER SERVING: CALORIES 293; PROTEIN 23g; CARBOHYDRATES 51g; TOTAL FAT 2.7g; SATURATED FAT 0.5g; CHOLESTEROL 34.2mg; SODIUM 140mg; FIBER 6.2g; BETA-CAROTENE 5,565ug; VITAMIN C 62mg; CALCIUM 166mg; IRON 3.3mg; FOLATE 128ug; MAGNESIUM 133mg; ZINC 1.7mg; SELENIUM 25.8ug

Black Bean Turkey Burgers 🌿

INGREDIENTS

1½ cups cooked black beans* or 1 (15-ounce) can no-salt-added or low-sodium black beans

8 ounces ground turkey breast

⅓ cup no-salt-added tomato sauce

10-ounce package frozen, chopped spinach, defrosted and excess water squeezed out

⅓ cup dry bread crumbs

⅓ cup finely chopped onion

2 tablespoons chopped fresh cilantro

1 teaspoon cumin

1 teaspoon chili powder

* Use ½ cup dried beans; see cooking instructions on page 19.

DIRECTIONS

Preheat the oven to 350°F.

Mash beans with a fork or potato masher. Stir in other ingredients.

Form into 4 patties. Bake for 30 minutes or until cooked through, turning once.

PER SERVING: CALORIES 240; PROTEIN 20.2g; CARBOHYDRATES 27g; TOTAL FAT 6.2g; SATURATED FAT 1.5g; CHOLESTEROL 44.8mg; SODIUM 281mg; FIBER 9g; BETA-CAROTENE 5,111ug; VITAMIN C 20mg; CALCIUM 163mg; IRON 4.2mg; FOLATE 208ug; MAGNESIUM 117mg; ZINC 2.3mg; SELENIUM 18.5ug

DESSERTS

*Recipes recommended for aggressive weight-loss
and diabetic diets and for people
with metabolic syndrome are marked with 🌿.*

DESSERTS

One trick to help prevent overeating is to have a delicious dessert at the conclusion of dinner—before you've overeaten. Let dessert mark the end of your day's eating experience and do not eat again until breakfast the next morning.

Fruit is a perfect dessert, either by itself or as part of a recipe. Always make sure your fruit is ripe and at the peak of perfection when you eat it. Take advantage of local seasonal produce. It will be fresher, tastier, and less expensive.

Stick to natural whole foods as sweeteners. I use fresh or frozen fruit or dried fruit to sweeten my desserts. If you are using dried fruit such as dates or raisins in your recipes, use just enough to make the dish moderately sweet. Make sure the dried fruit you use is unsulfured. I do not recommend agave or honey. They are concentrated sweeteners with minimal nutritional value. Avoid artificial sweeteners such as aspartame, saccharin, and sucralose; their safety is questionable.

The delicious fruit sorbets and ice "creams" included in this cookbook are made using a high-powered blender. They are quick and easy to make and healthfully satisfy your sweet tooth. You can start with my recipes and then get creative and put together your own favorite combinations. The frozen creations that contain nuts will stay softer and can be stored in the freezer before serving. This is because the fat content of the nuts helps to prevent the dessert from freezing solid. The sorbets that do not contain nuts should be eaten right after they are made. If they are stored in the freezer, they will become very hard.

I have also included some of my favorite decadent and nutrient-rich cakes, cookies, and pies. When you are in the mood for a fancy dessert or when you are bringing a special dish to a party, these scrumptious desserts are proof that you don't have to sacrifice taste and pleasure to eat healthfully.

Experiment with different varieties of a particular fruit.

There are many different types of apples, for instance, and they all have different flavors and textures. Enjoy Fuji, Honeycrisp, Pink Lady, Cameo, Braeburn, Empire, McIntosh, Jonagold, Granny Smith, and Golden Delicious both raw and cooked. Red Delicious is better eaten raw, not cooked. There is also a wide variety of pears. Anjou, Bartlett, and Comice are great for salads while Bosc and Seckel pears are for both eating and cooking.

Apple Berrynut Bites

SERVES 12

INGREDIENTS

- 2 cups unsulfured dried apples
- 1½ cups unsweetened vanilla soy, hemp, or almond milk
- 2 cups sliced fresh, organic strawberries (or frozen, thawed), divided
- ¼ cup oatmeal
- ½ cup raw pecans
- ½ cup raw Brazil nuts
- 3 tablespoons ground chia seeds
- 1 cup organic baby spinach
- ¼ cup unsweetened, shredded coconut, plus extra for garnish
- ½ tablespoon cinnamon
- ¼ teaspoon nutmeg
- ¾ cup dates, pitted

DIRECTIONS

Preheat the oven to 300°F.

Soak dried apples in soy milk for at least 1 hour or overnight.

In a high-powered blender, blend soaked apples, soy milk, and half the strawberries with remaining ingredients until smooth. Add a little more soy milk if needed.

Spoon into small muffin cups or small, oven-proof, custard cups and bake for 20 minutes.

Place 1 to 2 strawberry slices on top of each and sprinkle with additional coconut. Chill in the refrigerator before serving.

PER SERVING: CALORIES 190; PROTEIN 4g; CARBOHYDRATES 26g; TOTAL FAT 9.7g; SATURATED FAT 2g; SODIUM 19mg; FIBER 5.8g; BETA-CAROTENE 154ug; VITAMIN C 16mg; CALCIUM 61mg; IRON 1.6mg; FOLATE 20ug; MAGNESIUM 49mg; ZINC 0.8mg; SELENIUM 113ug

Chia Cookies 🌿

INGREDIENTS

- 1 cup currants
- 2 cups finely ground rolled oats
- ½ cup dried, unsweetened, shredded coconut
- 1 tablespoon ground chia seeds (see Note)
- 1 tablespoon whole chia seeds
- 1 teaspoon cinnamon
- 2 tablespoons raw almond butter
- ¾ cup unsweetened applesauce
- 1 teaspoon vanilla

DIRECTIONS

Preheat the oven to 200°F.

Soak ½ cup of the currants in ½ cup water for at least 1 hour.

Combine the ground oats, coconut, remaining currants, ground and whole chia seeds, and cinnamon in a bowl.

Place the almond butter, soaked currants and their soaking water, applesauce, and vanilla in a food processor. Blend until smooth, then add to the dry ingredients and mix well.

Form cookies using 2 teaspoons of dough per cookie. Place on a baking sheet lightly wiped with oil or covered with parchment paper. Bake for 90 minutes to 2 hours.

For diabetic, weight-loss, or metabolic syndrome diets, limit serving size to 1 cookie.

NOTE: Grind chia seeds in a high-powered blender or coffee grinder. Make a batch and store in the freezer.

PER COOKIE: CALORIES 79; PROTEIN 2g; CARBOHYDRATES 13g; TOTAL FAT 2.8g; SATURATED FAT 0.9g; SODIUM 7mg; FIBER 2g; BETA-CAROTENE 4ug; VITAMIN C 1mg; CALCIUM 20mg; IRON 0.8mg; FOLATE 7ug; MAGNESIUM 31mg; ZINC 0.4mg; SELENIUM 3.2ug

Goji Berry Walnut Squares with Chocolate Drizzle

>> Talia Fuhrman

These brownies are delightfully sweet, yet pack a hefty nutrient punch with the goji berries, nuts, oats, and dark chocolate. It's amazing how all of these ingredients come together to create the perfect treat.

SERVES 15

INGREDIENTS

1½ cups oats

1 cup walnuts

1 cup raw almonds or 1 cup almond flour (see Note)

1 teaspoon cinnamon

¾ cup chopped dates

½ cup water

1 banana

1 tablespoon vanilla extract

½ cup goji berries

2 ounces unsweetened dark chocolate

DIRECTIONS

In a high-powered blender, blend the oats until a flour forms. Add to a large bowl. Repeat process for the walnuts and almonds, being sure not to overprocess them as you don't want the oils to release. Add to the bowl and gently break apart any clumps with your fingers. It's okay if a few walnut or almond pieces remain. Stir in the cInnamon.

Add dates and water to blender and process until a slurry forms. Add banana and blend until well combined. Add date mixture to dry ingredients and mix until no flour remains. Stir in vanilla and goji berries.

Line an 8-inch square pan with aluminum foil or parchment paper. Scoop the dough into the pan. Dip a knife in water and spread dough until smooth. Place in the freezer for 30 minutes.

Place the unsweetened chocolate in a microwave-proof bowl and heat in the microwave for 1 minute, stir, and heat for another 30 seconds or until completely melted. Remove pan from freezer. Using a small spoon, drizzle with chocolate to add a decorative touch. Cut into squares.

Store in the freezer for a guilt-free snack. They can be eaten straight from the freezer or heated in the microwave for 30 to 45 seconds.

NOTE: Almond flour is simply raw, whole almonds that have been ground into a fine powder. It can be purchased in health food stores and many supermarkets but it is best to grind almonds and make it fresh.

PER SERVING: CALORIES 233; PROTEIN 7g; CARBOHYDRATES 26g; TOTAL FAT 13.1g; SATURATED FAT 2.3g; SODIUM 16mg; FIBER 5g; BETA-CAROTENE 5ug; VITAMIN C 11mg; CALCIUM 47mg; IRON 2.6mg; FOLATE 24ug; MAGNESIUM 86mg; ZINC 1.6mg; SELENIUM 5.3ug

Sweet Potato Peanut Cookies

>> Talia Fuhrman

MAKES 12 COOKIES

INGREDIENTS

- 2 tablespoons ground chia or flax seeds
- 1½ cups cooked white beans or 1 (15-ounce) can no-salt-added or low-sodium white beans, drained
- 2 tablespoons natural, unsalted peanut butter
- 1–2 ripe bananas (second one is optional, to be added later in chunks, if desired)
- ½ cup baked and peeled sweet potato

- 6 Medjool or 12 regular (Deglet Noor) dates, pits removed
- 1 teaspoon cinnamon
- ½ teaspoon nutmeg
- 1 tablespoon vanilla extract
- 1 cup whole-wheat flour
- 1 teaspoon baking powder
- ½ cup unsulfured, dried apricots, sliced into small pieces

DIRECTIONS

Preheat the oven to 350°F. In a cup or small bowl, mix ground chia seeds with ½ cup water and stir. Let sit for 2 minutes to form a gel.

In a Vitamix or other high-powered blender, combine chia seed gel, white beans, peanut butter, 1 banana, sweet potato, dates, cinnamon, nutmeg, and vanilla extract. Blend until smooth and creamy.

In a large bowl, combine the whole-wheat flour and baking powder and mix thoroughly. Add the blended mixture to this dry mixture and mix until flour is totally combined. Stir in apricot slices and thin slices of banana and mix.

Place parchment paper on a large cookie sheet or coat sheet with a thin layer of cooking spray. Drop batter by spoonfuls onto the sheet and bake for 20 minutes.

PER COOKIE: CALORIES 171; PROTEIN 5g; CARBOHYDRATES 33g; TOTAL FAT 3.3g; SATURATED FAT 1.1g; SODIUM 7mg; FIBER 5.2g; BETA-CAROTENE 1,090ug; VITAMIN C 3mg; CALCIUM 64mg; IRON 1.9mg; FOLATE 31ug; MAGNESIUM 54mg; ZINC 0.9mg; SELENIUM 8.2ug

Fudgy Black Bean Brownies

MAKES 16 SQUARES

INGREDIENTS

2 cups cooked black beans* or canned, no-salt-added or low-sodium black beans, drained

1¼ cups dates, pitted

2 tablespoons raw almond butter

1 teaspoon vanilla

½ cup natural, nonalkalized cocoa powder

1 tablespoon ground chia seeds

* Use ⅔ cup dried beans; see cooking instructions on page 19.

DIRECTIONS

Preheat the oven to 200°F.

Combine the black beans, dates, almond butter, and vanilla in a food processor or high-powered blender. Blend until smooth. Add the remaining ingredients and blend again. Pour into a very lightly oiled 8×8-inch baking pan. Bake for 90 minutes. Cool completely before cutting into small squares.

NOTE: These brownies can be stored in a covered container in the refrigerator for up to one week. For an added treat, serve with a dollop of Avocado Chocolate Pudding (page 296) on top.

PER SERVING: CALORIES 94; PROTEIN 3g; CARBOHYDRATES 19g; TOTAL FAT 1.9g; SATURATED FAT 0.4g; SODIUM 1mg; FIBER 4.2g; BETA-CAROTENE 13ug; CALCIUM 30mg; IRON 1.1mg; FOLATE 37ug; MAGNESIUM 43mg; ZINC 0.6mg; SELENIUM 0.6ug

Banana Oat Bars

SERVES 8

INGREDIENTS

2 cups quick-cooking rolled oats (not instant)

½ cup shredded coconut

½ cup raisins or chopped pitted dates

¼ cup chopped walnuts

2 large ripe bananas, mashed

¾ cup finely chopped apple

2 tablespoons ground flax seeds

DIRECTIONS

Preheat the oven to 350°F. Mix all the ingredients in a large bowl until well combined. Press into a 9 x 9-inch baking pan and bake for 30 minutes. Cool on a wire rack. When cool, cut into squares or bars.

NOTE: For Banana Oat Spice Bars, mix in:
½ teaspoon ground cinnamon
¼ teaspoon allspice
¼ teaspoon ground cloves
¼ teaspoon ground nutmeg
⅛ teaspoon black pepper

PER SERVING: CALORIES 247; PROTEIN 8g; CARBOHYDRATES 41g; TOTAL FAT 6.9g; SATURATED FAT 2.2g; SODIUM 3mg; FIBER 5.9g; BETA-CAROTENE 8ug; VITAMIN C 3mg; CALCIUM 31mg; IRON 2.3mg; FOLATE 33ug; MAGNESIUM 87mg; ZINC 1.8mg; SELENIUM 11ug

Cara's Apple Strudel 🌿

INGREDIENTS

- ½ cup vanilla soy, hemp, or almond milk
- ¾ teaspoon vanilla extract
- 1 teaspoon cinnamon
- 3 apples, peeled, cored, and chopped
- ¼ cup raisins, chopped
- ½ cup old-fashioned rolled oats
- ¼ cup ground raw walnuts
- 2 tablespoons ground flax seeds

DIRECTIONS

Preheat the oven to 350°F. In a bowl, mix the milk, vanilla, and cinnamon until combined. Stir in the chopped apples, raisins, oats, ground walnuts, and flax seeds.

Pour into an 8×8-inch baking dish. Bake uncovered for 1 hour.

PER SERVING: CALORIES 190; PROTEIN 7g; CARBOHYDRATES 33g; TOTAL FAT 5.9g; SATURATED FAT 0.5g; SODIUM 14mg; FIBER 5.3g; BETA-CAROTENE 84ug; VITAMIN C 5mg; CALCIUM 44mg; IRON 1.5mg; FOLATE 13ug; MAGNESIUM 65mg; ZINC 0.7mg; SELENIUM 4.4ug

Healthy Chocolate Cake

SERVES 16

INGREDIENTS

. . . .

FOR THE CAKE:

1⅔ cups whole-wheat flour

1 teaspoon baking powder

3 teaspoons baking soda

3½ cups pitted dates, divided

1 cup pineapple chunks in own juice, drained

1 banana

1 cup unsweetened applesauce

1 cup shredded beets

¾ cup shredded carrots

½ cup shredded zucchini

4 tablespoons natural cocoa powder

½ cup currants

1 cup chopped walnuts

1½ cups water

2 teaspoons vanilla extract

FOR THE CHOCOLATE NUT ICING:

1 cup raw macadamia nuts or raw cashews, unsalted

1 cup vanilla soy, hemp, or almond milk

⅔ cup pitted dates

⅓ cup Brazil nuts or hazelnuts

2 tablespoons natural cocoa powder

1 teaspoon vanilla extract

DIRECTIONS

Preheat the oven to 350°F.

Mix flour, baking powder, and baking soda in a small bowl. Set aside.

In a blender or food processor (see Note), puree 3 cups of the dates, pineapple, banana, and applesauce.

Slice remaining ½ cup dates into ½-inch-thick pieces. In a large bowl, mix sliced dates, beets, carrots, zucchini, cocoa powder, currants, walnuts, water, vanilla, and flour mixture.

Add the blended mixture and mix well. Spread in a 9½ x 13½-inch nonstick baking pan.

Bake for 1 hour or until a toothpick inserted into the center comes out clean.

To make individual servings, bake in muffin pans lined with paper liners. Reduce cooking time to 20 to 25 minutes.

For the chocolate nut icing, combine all ingredients in a high-powered blender (see Note) until smooth and creamy. Place a dollop over warm cake and serve or spread on cooled cake.

NOTE: A food processor may be used, but the icing will not be as smooth.

PER SERVING: CALORIES 341; PROTEIN 7g; CARBOHYDRATES 61g; TOTAL FAT 11g; SATURATED FAT 1.5g; SODIUM 260mg; FIBER 8.1g; BETA-CAROTENE 447ug; VITAMIN C 4mg; CALCIUM 65mg; IRON 2.6mg; FOLATE 45ug; MAGNESIUM 99mg; ZINC 2mg; SELENIUM 13ug

Coconut Carrot Cream Pie

SERVES 8

INGREDIENTS

FOR THE FILLING:

1 cup unsulfured dried apples, chopped

⅓ cup unsulfured dried apricots

½ cup muscat or other sweet dessert wine

3 apples, grated

⅓ cup raisins

¼ cup walnuts

1½ cups shredded carrot

½ cup shredded zucchini

½ cup shredded beet

½ cup unsweetened, shredded coconut

¾ teaspoon cinnamon

¼ teaspoon nutmeg

FOR THE PIE CRUST:

⅓ cup old-fashioned oats, ground

1 cup raw almonds

1 cup pitted dates

1 tablespoon chia seed gel (see Note)

FOR THE TOPPING:

2 vanilla beans, split lengthwise

1⅓ cup macadamia nuts

1 cup soy, hemp, or almond milk

⅔ cup pitted dates

DIRECTIONS

To make the filling, marinate the chopped dry apples and apricots in wine overnight in the refrigerator or for 1 hour at room temperature.

Combine grated apples, raisins, and walnuts in a food processor or blender, then add in the soaked, dried fruit/wine mixture and process until combined. Drain and press excess moisture from carrots, zucchini, and beets and mix into apple mixture along with coconut, cinnamon, and nutmeg.

To make the pie crust, place almonds and oats in a food processor and process until very finely ground. Add dates and process until chopped and mixed well. Add chia seed gel and pulse to mix in. Press mixture into a pie plate to form shell. (More chia seed gel may be added if mixture is too dry.)

To make the topping, scrape seeds from vanilla bean with a dull knife and add to a food processor or high-powered blender along with nuts, nondairy milk, and dates. Blend until smooth and creamy.

Add filling to pie crust and spread on topping. Refrigerate until ready to serve.

NOTE: To make chia seed gel, mix 3 tablespoons chia seeds in ¾ cup water and let stand for at least 15 minutes. Process in food processor to make into a paste.

PER SERVING: CALORIES 354; PROTEIN 8g; CARBOHYDRATES 52g; TOTAL FAT 14.4g; SATURATED FAT 2.6g; SODIUM 42mg; FIBER 9.2g; BETA-CAROTENE 2,039ug; VITAMIN C 7mg; CALCIUM 88mg; IRON 2.2mg; FOLATE 36ug; MAGNESIUM 93mg; ZINC 1.2mg; SELENIUM 3.5ug

Pumpkin Pie with Almond Crust

SERVES 10

INGREDIENTS

FOR THE PIE CRUST:

1 cup raw almonds

1 teaspoon ground chia seeds

1 cup pitted dates

2 teaspoons water

FOR THE FILLING:

1 (15-ounce) can pumpkin

½ cup pitted dates, soaked in ¼ cup water

½ cup raisins

1 teaspoon ground cinnamon

½ teaspoon ground ginger

½ teaspoon ground nutmeg

2½ tablespoons arrowroot powder

1 10-ounce package soft tofu

FOR THE CASHEW CREAM TOPPING:

1⅓ cups raw cashews

¾ cup vanilla soy, hemp, or almond milk

⅔ cup pitted dates

DIRECTIONS

Preheat the oven to 350°F.

To make the crust, combine the raw almonds and 1 teaspoon ground chia seeds in a food processor. Pulse until finely ground. Add the dates and water and process until the mixture gathers into a ball. Press the mixture into a very lightly oiled 8-inch pie plate. Pre-bake the crust for 5 minutes.

To make the filling, blend the pumpkin, dates, and soaking water in a high-powered blender. Add the raisins, spices, arrowroot powder and tofu. Blend until smooth. Pour mixture into prebaked pie shell. Cover with aluminum foil and bake for 60 minutes. Uncover and continue baking an additional 15 minutes. Pie filling will firm up as it cools.

While pie is in the oven, make the Cashew Cream Topping. Blend all ingredients together in a high-powered blender.

Serve with a dollop of Cashew Cream.

PER SERVING: CALORIES 337; PROTEIN 7g; CARBOHYDRATES 51g; TOTAL FAT 14g; SATURATED FAT 2g; SODIUM 21mg; FIBER 5g; BETA-CAROTENE 1,386ug; VITAMIN C 4mg; CALCIUM 97mg; IRON 3.2mg; FOLATE 46ug; MAGNESIUM 108mg; ZINC 1.9mg; SELENIUM 7.4ug

Pineapple Strawbana Pie

SERVES 8

INGREDIENTS

FOR THE PIE SHELL:

1 cup almonds

1 cup walnuts

⅓ cup pitted dates

1 apple, cored, peeled, and cut in chunks

FOR THE PIE FILLING:

5 bananas, 3 sliced and 2 frozen (see Note)

3 kiwis, sliced

½ fresh pineapple, chopped

6 ounces frozen strawberries, slightly thawed and sliced

½ cup soy, hemp, or almond milk

DIRECTIONS

Make the pie shell by placing the nuts and dates in a food processor and chopping well. Add apple and process until a fine texture. Press into a pie plate to shape a crust.

For the pie filling, place the sliced bananas on the crust, pressing slightly. Place kiwis and pineapple on top of bananas.

Add frozen bananas, strawberries, and soy milk to a blender and blend until smooth. Pour over fruit, cover, and freeze for at least 2 hours before serving. Remove from freezer before serving to allow the pie to thaw slightly.

NOTE: Freeze 2 of the bananas at least 12 hours ahead of time.

PER SERVING: CALORIES 316; PROTEIN 8g; CARBOHYDRATES 34g; TOTAL FAT 19.5g; SATURATED FAT 1.7g; SODIUM 16mg; FIBER 6.7g; BETA-CAROTENE 107ug; VITAMIN C 53mg; CALCIUM 80mg; IRON 1.8mg; FOLATE 52ug; MAGNESIUM 108mg; ZINC 1.3mg; SELENIUM 2.9ug

No-Bake Key Lime Pie

If you can't find Key limes, use regular limes.

SERVES 12

INGREDIENTS

- ⅔ cup raw walnuts
- ⅔ cup unsweetened, shredded coconut
- ⅔ cup old-fashioned rolled oats
- 20 pitted Medjool dates, divided (4 for crust, 16 for filling)
- 3 avocados
- ¾ cup fresh Key lime juice (approximately 1½ pounds of Key limes)
- ¼ cup raw cashew butter

DIRECTIONS

To make the crust, grind the walnuts, coconut, and oats in a food processor, using the S-blade. Add 4 of the dates and continue to process until the mixture starts to hold together. Press into a 9-inch pie plate.

To make the filling, combine the remaining dates with the avocados, lime juice, and cashew butter in a high-powered blender and blend until smooth. Pour into crust and refrigerate for at least 4 hours before serving.

PER SERVING: CALORIES 312; PROTEIN 5g; CARBOHYDRATES 43g; TOTAL FAT 16.4g; SATURATED FAT 3.8g; SODIUM 4mg; FIBER 8.4g; BETA-CAROTENE 81ug; VITAMIN C 18mg; CALCIUM 45mg; IRON 1.3mg; FOLATE 47ug; MAGNESIUM 79mg; ZINC 1.2mg; SELENIUM 2.9ug

Mango Pudding 🌿

INGREDIENTS

- ¼ cup raw almonds
- 2 ripe mangoes, peeled and cut into pieces
- 1 banana
- 3 dates, pitted
- ⅛ cup unsweetened, shredded coconut
- ½ teaspoon vanilla
- ¼ cup currants
- ⅛ teaspoon cinnamon

DIRECTIONS

Grind almonds in a high-powered blender and then add mangoes, banana, dates, coconut, and vanilla and blend until smooth and creamy.

Place in a bowl, stir in currants, and sprinkle with cinnamon.

Chill for at least 2 hours before serving.

PER SERVING: CALORIES 266; PROTEIN 5g; CARBOHYDRATES 51g; TOTAL FAT 7.8g; SATURATED FAT 1.6g; SODIUM 8mg; FIBER 6.6g; BETA-CAROTENE 631ug; VITAMIN C 42mg; CALCIUM 57mg; IRON 1.3mg; FOLATE 34ug; MAGNESIUM 66mg; ZINC 0.6mg; SELENIUM 2.2ug

Persimmon Pudding 🍃

» Chef James Rohrbacher

SERVES 6

INGREDIENTS

½ cup Dr. Fuhrman's Mangosteen Vinegar

1 cup water

2 teaspoons arrowroot powder, dissolved in an additional ¼ cup cold water

8 very ripe Hachiya persimmons, stem removed, unpeeled (see Note)

DIRECTIONS

Bring vinegar and the cup of water to a boil in a small saucepan. Once boiling, whisk in the arrowroot/cold water mixture and let boil for 2 minutes, but no longer, whisking occasionally. Remove from heat and cool.

In a high-powered blender, puree persimmons and ½ cup of the vinegar mixture (vinaigrette) until it reaches the consistency of a salad dressing.

Pour into small bowls, cover with plastic wrap, and chill. For a more elegant presentation, pour into champagne, cordial, or martini glasses, cover with plastic wrap, and chill. The pudding will firm up if chilled overnight.

If desired, pudding can be served with a dollop of Cashew Cream Topping: blend 1⅓ cups raw cashews; ¾ cup soy, hemp, or almond milk; and ⅔ cup pitted dates together in a high-powered blender.

NOTE: Hachiya persimmons should be eaten when very ripe (completely soft even at the bottom edge). The fruit has a high tannin content, which makes the immature fruit very astringent. The tannin gradually disappears as the fruit matures. When ready to eat, the flesh becomes sweet, aromatic, and almost liquid. A ripe persimmon is like a thin skin full of thick jelly.

PER SERVING: CALORIES 161; PROTEIN 1.3g; CARBOHYDRATES 42g; TOTAL FAT 0.4g; SATURATED FAT 0g; SODIUM 5mg; FIBER 8g; BETA-CAROTENE 567ug; VITAMIN C 17mg; CALCIUM 21mg; IRON 0.4mg; FOLATE 21ug; MAGNESIUM 22mg; ZINC 0.3mg; SELENIUM 1ug

Avocado Chocolate Pudding

This rich and creamy pudding is wonderful topped with a generous helping of fresh berries.

SERVES 4

INGREDIENTS

1 ripe avocado, peeled, pit removed

½–¾ cups soy, hemp, or almond milk (start with ½ cup and add more if needed to blend)

4 tablespoons natural, nonalkalized cocoa powder

6–10 dates, pitted (depending on size and sweetness)

½ teaspoon vanilla extract

DIRECTIONS

Blend all ingredients in a high-powered blender.

PER SERVING: CALORIES 199; PROTEIN 3g; CARBOHYDRATES 38g; TOTAL FAT 7.3g; SATURATED FAT 1.3g; SODIUM 5mg; FIBER 7.4g; BETA-CAROTENE 64ug; VITAMIN C 4mg; CALCIUM 39mg; IRON 1.3mg; FOLATE 46ug; MAGNESIUM 60mg; ZINC 0.8mg; SELENIUM 0.9ug

Berry "Yogurt" 🌿

May be served over fresh or frozen berries.

SERVES 2

INGREDIENTS

2 cups blueberries, blackberries, or strawberries, fresh or frozen

¾ cup soy, almond, or hemp milk

2 tablespoons ground flax or chia seeds

4 dates, pitted

DIRECTIONS

Add all ingredients to a high-powered blender and blend until smooth. Chill before serving.

PER SERVING: CALORIES 214; PROTEIN 25g; CARBOHYDRATES 42g; TOTAL FAT 5.2g; SATURATED FAT 0.5g; SODIUM 53mg; FIBER 7.9g; BETA-CAROTENE 378ug; VITAMIN C 14mg; CALCIUM 67mg; IRON 2mg; FOLATE 32ug; MAGNESIUM 66mg; ZINC 1mg; SELENIUM 6.7ug

Pomegranate Poached Pears with Chocolate and Raspberry Sauces

SERVES 6

INGREDIENTS

6 medium Bosc pears

2 cups pomegranate juice or red wine

1 whole cinnamon stick

6 whole cloves

2 tablespoons goji berries

FOR THE CHOCOLATE SAUCE:

1 cup frozen blueberries

1½ cups soy, hemp, or almond milk

1 cup pitted dates

⅔ cup raw macadamia nuts

1 tablespoon unsweetened, natural, nonalkalized cocoa, or more for a darker, stronger sauce

½ teaspoon vanilla extract

1 teaspoon turmeric (to adjust color)

FOR THE RASPBERRY SAUCE:

10 ounces frozen red raspberries (about 1½ cups), thawed

DIRECTIONS

Peel pears, leaving stems intact. Slice a little off the bottom of each pear so that they stand up. In a large saucepan, place pears standing up snugly together. Pour in pomegranate juice or wine. Add cinnamon, cloves, and goji berries. Gently simmer, covered, for about 20 minutes until pears are tender. Remove pears and refrigerate until ready to serve. Reduce poaching liquid until it becomes a syrup.

For the chocolate sauce, place blueberries, soy milk, dates, macadamia nuts, cocoa powder, vanilla, and turmeric in a blender. Blend until very smooth and creamy. Add more soy milk if needed.

For the raspberry sauce, place defrosted raspberries in a blender and blend until smooth. Push through sieve to remove seeds. Mix in poaching syrup.

Place a generous dollop of chocolate sauce on dessert plate. Place pear on chocolate and drizzle raspberry sauce over pear.

PER SERVING: CALORIES 296; PROTEIN 4g; CARBOHYDRATES 62g; TOTAL FAT 5.8g; SATURATED FAT 0.9g; SODIUM 29mg; FIBER 11.4g; BETA-CAROTENE 182ug; VITAMIN C 20mg; CALCIUM 56mg; IRON 1.6mg; FOLATE 33ug; MAGNESIUM 51mg; ZINC 0.7mg; SELENIUM 3ug

Banana Walnut Ice Cream

SERVES 2

INGREDIENTS

- 2 ripe bananas, frozen (see Note)
- ⅓ cup vanilla soy, hemp, or almond milk
- 2 tablespoons chopped walnuts
- ½ teaspoon vanilla extract or 1 vanilla bean (see box)

DIRECTIONS

Blend all ingredients together in a high-powered blender until smooth and creamy.

NOTE: Freeze ripe bananas at least 12 hours in advance. To freeze bananas, peel, cut in thirds, and wrap tightly in plastic wrap.

PER SERVING: CALORIES 174; PROTEIN 4g; CARBOHYDRATES 30g; TOTAL FAT 5.9g; SATURATED FAT 0.7g; SODIUM 23mg; FIBER 4.1g; BETA-CAROTENE 178ug; VITAMIN C 10mg; CALCIUM 28mg; IRON 1mg; FOLATE 37ug; MAGNESIUM 53mg; ZINC 0.6mg; SELENIUM 3.5ug

> Using a vanilla bean will add a subtle, yet complex flavor to this simple dessert. Split the vanilla bean lengthwise and scrape the inner gel-like lining from the bean using a dull knife.

Chocolate Cherry Ice Cream ✐

SERVES 2

INGREDIENTS

½ cup vanilla soy, hemp, or almond milk

2 tablespoons natural, nonalkalized cocoa powder

4 pitted dates

1½ cups dark sweet cherries, frozen

1 vanilla bean pod

DIRECTIONS

Blend all ingredients together in a high-powered blender or food processor until smooth and creamy. Split the vanilla bean lengthwise and roll open. Scrape out the paste and seeds inside the pod with a knife or spoon and add to blender. If using a regular blender, only add half the cherries, blend until smooth, then add remaining cherries and continue to blend.

NOTE: You can use frozen berries or banana instead of cherries. Freeze ripe bananas at least 12 hours in advance. To freeze bananas, peel, cut into thirds, and wrap tightly in plastic wrap.

PER SERVING: CALORIES 109; PROTEIN 4g; CARBOHYDRATES 23g; TOTAL FAT 1.7g; SATURATED FAT 0.4g; SODIUM 34mg; FIBER 4.1g; BETA-CAROTENE 263ug; VITAMIN C 8mg; CALCIUM 41mg; IRON 1.4mg; FOLATE 15ug; MAGNESIUM 41mg; ZINC 0.5mg; SELENIUM 3.3ug

Fuhrman Fudgesicles 🌿

SERVES 3

INGREDIENTS

. . . .

- 2 ripe bananas
- 1 cup raw cashews
- 3 tablespoons natural, nonalkalized cocoa powder
- ½ teaspoon vanilla extract or 2 vanilla bean interiors

DIRECTIONS

. . . .

Blend all ingredients together in a food processor or high-powered blender until smooth.

Spoon into an ice pop tray or ice cube tray and freeze for at least 2 hours before serving.

Rinse outside of trays with hot water to pull the pops out easily.

. . . .

PER SERVING: CALORIES 251; PROTEIN 7g; CARBOHYDRATES 24g; TOTAL FAT 16.6g; SATURATED FAT 3.5g; SODIUM 6mg; FIBER 3.5g; BETA-CAROTENE 15ug; VITAMIN C 5mg; CALCIUM 22mg; IRON 2.3mg; FOLATE 35ug; MAGNESIUM 119mg; ZINC 2mg; SELENIUM 4.8ug

Peach Apricot Sorbet 🌿

INGREDIENTS

· ·

2 cups frozen peaches

¼ cup soy, hemp, or almond milk or water

4 unsweetened and unsulfured dried apricots, chopped

DIRECTIONS

· ·

Blend all ingredients in a high-powered blender.

· ·

PER SERVING: CALORIES 92; PROTEIN 3g; CARBOHYDRATES 20g; TOTAL FAT 1g; SATURATED FAT 0.1g; SODIUM 17mg; FIBER 3g; BETA-CAROTENE 511ug; VITAMIN C 10mg; CALCIUM 24mg; IRON 0.9mg; FOLATE 12ug; MAGNESIUM 24mg; ZINC 0.4mg; SELENIUM 1.7ug

Strawberry Pineapple Sorbet 🍃

SERVES 2

INGREDIENTS

....

4 slices unsweetened and unsulfured dried pineapple

½ cup orange juice

1 (10-ounce) bag frozen strawberries

1 cup sliced fresh, organic strawberries, optional

DIRECTIONS

....

Soak dried pineapple in orange juice for a few hours or overnight. Chop dried pineapple, add to a high-powered blender along with frozen strawberries, and blend until smooth.

Blend all ingredients, except fresh strawberries, in a high-powered blender.

Pour into sorbet glasses and, if desired, top with sliced, fresh strawberries.

....

PER SERVING: CALORIES 150; PROTEIN 2g; CARBOHYDRATES 38g; TOTAL FAT 0.5g; SODIUM 12mg; FIBER 4.9g; BETA-CAROTENE 64ug; VITAMIN C 132mg; CALCIUM 49mg; IRON 1.5mg; FOLATE 60ug; MAGNESIUM 32mg; ZINC 0.3mg; SELENIUM 1.3ug

Red Velvet Sorbet 🌿

SERVES 4

INGREDIENTS

- 4 large ripe bananas, frozen (see Note)
- 10 ounces frozen raspberries
- 2 tablespoons natural, nonalkalized cocoa powder
- 4–5 pitted dates, chopped

DIRECTIONS

Blend all ingredients in a high-powered blender untll creamy. Refreeze briefly (3 to 5 minutes).

If desired, top with Pecan Cream. To make Pecan Cream, blend ⅔ cup pecans; ½ cup soy, hemp, or almond milk; and 4 or 5 pitted dates in a high-powered blender.

NOTE: *Freeze ripe bananas at least 12 hours in advance. To freeze bananas, peel, cut in thirds, and wrap tightly in plastic wrap.*

PER SERVING: CALORIES 171; PROTEIN 3g; CARBOHYDRATES 43g; TOTAL FAT 1.2g; SATURATED FAT 0.4g; SODIUM 3mg; FIBER 9.2g; BETA-CAROTENE 40ug; VITAMIN C 29mg; CALCIUM 30mg; IRON 1.2mg; FOLATE 41ug; MAGNESIUM 63mg; ZINC 0.7mg; SELENIUM 1.9ug

Chocolate Dip

SERVES 10

INGREDIENTS

2 cups organic baby spinach

1½ cups soy, hemp, or almond milk

1 cup frozen blueberries

1 cup pitted dates

⅔ cup raw almonds

2 generous tablespoons natural, nonalkalized cocoa powder

½ teaspoon vanilla extract

DIRECTIONS

Place all ingredients in a high-powered blender. Blend until very smooth and creamy.

Serve with a variety of fresh fruit.

PER SERVING: CALORIES 137; PROTEIN 5g; CARBOHYDRATES 20g; TOTAL FAT 5.9g; SATURATED FAT 0.6g; SODIUM 28mg; FIBER 3.8g; BETA-CAROTENE 475ug; VITAMIN C 2mg; CALCIUM 50mg; IRON 1.3mg; FOLATE 25ug; MAGNESIUM 54mg; ZINC 1mg; SELENIUM 2.7ug

EAT TO LIVE FOR ALL OCCASIONS

Here are some nutritarian menus for everyday and special occasions. Try these combinations and put together your own to create great-tasting, memorable meals.

WEEKDAY BREAKFAST

Quick Banana Berry Breakfast To Go *(page 65)*

Super Easy Blended Salad *(page 51)*

LEISURELY BRUNCH

Butternut Breakfast Soup *(page 69)*

Tuscan Tofu Scramble *(page 72)*

Mixed berries with ground hemp or chia seeds

BROWN BAG LUNCH

Italian Stuffer *(page 258)*

Orange Sesame Micro Salad *(page 118)*

Apple or other fresh fruit

SOUP AND SALAD CLASSIC LUNCH

Cream of Asparagus Soup *(page 152)*

Chopped Romaine lettuce with Nutritarian Caesar
Dressing *(page 82)*

Melon or other fresh fruit

FESTIVE LUNCHEON

Raw vegetables with Mushroom Walnut Pâté *(page 101)*

Lemon Cauliflower Risotto *(page 221)*

Orange Zest Chard *(page 214)*

Chocolate Cherry Ice Cream *(page 301)*

CASUAL BACKYARD DINNER

Raw vegetables with Tuscan White Bean Dip *(page 100)*

Better Burgers *(page 250)*

Corn on the cob

Super Slaw *(page 119)*

Watermelon

MEXICAN FIESTA

Mixed greens with Guacamole Dressing *(page 92)*

Bean Enchiladas *(page 254)*

Fresh Tomato Salsa *(page 96)*

Sliced mango

ITALIAN DINNER PARTY

Tuscan Cannellini Bean Soup with a Chiffonade of
   Collard Greens *(page 170)*
Spinach and arugula salad with Almond Balsamic
   Vinaigrette *(page 81)*
Eggplant Cannelloni with Pine Nut Romesco Sauce *(page 194)*
Strawberry Pineapple Sorbet *(page 304)*

QUICK AND EASY DINNER

Boston lettuce salad with Russian Fig Dressing *(page 91)*
Goji Chili Stew *(page 177)*
Blueberries or other fresh fruit

SUNDAY FAMILY DINNER

Dr. Fuhrman's Famous Anticancer Soup *(page 154)*
Acorn Squash Supreme *(page 232)*
California Creamed Kale *(page 211)*
Healthy Chocolate Cake *(page 286)*

STIR-FRY CLASSIC

Mixed greens and watercress with Ginger Almond
   Dressing *(page 86)*
Asian Vegetable Stir-Fry *(page 182)*
Persimmons or other fresh fruit

ACKNOWLEDGMENTS

I would like to thank all the people whose creativity and culinary talent made this book possible. What makes this book extra special is the wonderful bonus recipes that came from a variety of nutritarian cooks and chefs mentioned below. The inclusion of these contributions demonstrates the growing excitement and popularity of nutritarian cuisine. There is no reason why the healthiest foods cannot be prepared deliciously, as indicated by the thousands of creative professionals who have already jumped on board.

Some recipes were contributed by people belonging to my member center at DrFuhrman.com: among them Rich Amiot, Claudia Bullock, Laura King, Debbie Warne-Jackson, Krista Schroeder, and Carol Davis-Hawkins. Special thanks to a talented group of professional chefs, who not only contributed some of their recipes to this publication, but whose careers promote the culinary possibilities of a nutritarian diet. These chefs include Martin Oswald, James Rohrbacher, Jack Hunt, Paul Bogardus, Christine Waltermyer, and my daughter, Talia Fuhrman.

I would like to thank my team at DrFuhrman.com who contributed their efforts to the completion of this book, especially Janice Marra, Linda Popescu, and Lisa Fuhrman. They have been essential to compiling this collection of recipes and helping me translate the principles of eating a nutrient-dense plant-based diet into a reality for the many people who wish to adopt this lifestyle.

I would also like to acknowledge Robyn Rolfes, of Creative Syndicate, for the design work that went into putting this book together. And, of course, the wonderful people at HarperOne, especially Gideon Weil and Melinda Mullin for their devotion to getting this message out as a mission to better humanity and see it as more than just a job. I am grateful for the opportunity to work with them.

INDEX

tip on, 157; Slow Cooker Eggplant Breakfast, 68; Too-Busy-To-Cook Vegetable Bean Soup, 168. *See also specific recipes*

carrots: ANDI score of, 28; herbs and spices to enhance flavor of, 180; Red Quinoa, Roasted Rainbow Carrots, Brussels Sprouts, Pearl Onions, and Dulse Salad with Pumpkin Seeds and Verjus, 242–243; as super food, 29. *See also specific recipes*

cashews: ANDI score of, 28; as super food, 29

casual backyard dinner, 308

cauliflower: ANDI score of, 28; as anticancer food, 159; Cauliflower and Green Pea Curry, 219; Cauliflower Spinach Mashed "Potatoes," 220; for dipping, 94; herbs and spices to enhance flavor of, 180; Lemon Cauliflower Risotto, 221, 308; recommended preparation of, 8–9; as super food, 29; Veg-Head Bean Burrito, 255. *See also specific recipes*

cayenne pepper flavor, 36

celery "Dirty Dozen" pesticide level, 39

celery seeds, 37

cheddar cheese ANDI score, 28

cherimoya, 15

cherries: ANDI score of, 28; Chocolate Cherry Ice Cream, 301, 308; Chocolate Cherry Smoothie, 52; Polenta with Wilted Greens, Roasted Portobello Mushrooms and Black Cherry Vinaigrette, 230–231

cherry tomatoes, 94. *See also* tomatoes

chia seeds: Chia Cookies, 278–279; as high-omega–3 fats source, 20–23; as super food, 29. *See also specific recipes*

chicken: ANDI score of chicken breast, 28; Creole Chicken and Spinach, 273

chickpeas. *See* garbanzo beans (chickpeas)

chicory and frisée (curly endive), 112

chiffonade technique, 171

chili powder flavor, 36

chip recipes: Kale Krinkle Chips, 104; Pita/Tortilla Crisps, 103; recommended for weight-loss, diabetic, and metabolic syndrome, 93

chives flavor, 36

chocolate: Avocado Chocolate Pudding, 296; Chocolate Cherry Smoothie, 52; Goji Berry Walnut Squares with Chocolate Drizzle, 280–281; Healthy Chocolate Cake, 286–287, 309; Pomegranate Poached Pears with Chocolate and Raspberry Sauces, 298–299; Sweet Potato Peanut Chocolate Chip Cookies, 282. *See also* cocoa powder

cholesterol-lowering foods, 84

Choose My Plate, 30

cilantro flavor, 36

cinnamon flavor, 36

"Clean Fifteen" produce, 39

cloves flavor, 36

cocoa bean flavanols, 52

cocoa powder: Chocolate Cherry Ice Cream, 301, 308; Chocolate Cherry Smoothie, 52; Chocolate Dip, 306; Fudgy Black Bean Brownies, 283; Fuhrman Fudgesicles, 302; Healthy Chocolate Cake, 286–287, 309; phytonutrients and antioxidants in, 52; production of, 52; Red Velvet Sorbet, 305. *See also* chocolate

cola: ANDI score of, 28; nutritarian guideline on avoiding, 5

collard greens: ANDI score of, 28; as anticancer food, 159; Collard Dijon Wraps, 263; recommended preparation of, 8–9; recommended steaming times for, 10; as super food, 29

cooked vegetables, dipping, 94

cookies. *See* dessert recipes

Cooking to Live: food shopping, 37–38; getting rid of food addictions, 40; helpful tools and techniques, 33–34; make a weekly plan, 39–40; should I buy organic produce?, 38–39; spices, herbs, and condiments, 35–37. *See also* Eat to Live; nutritarian tips

coriander seeds, 110

corn: ANDI score of, 28; "Clean Fifteen" pesticide level of sweet, 39; on the cob, 308; herbs and spices to enhance flavor of, 180; as one of the Native American "three sisters," 167; Summer Corn and Tomato Sauté, 225; Too-Busy-To-Cook Vegetable Bean Soup, 168

cornbread, 266

corn chips ANDI score, 28

cornmeal, 73

coronary heart disease, 84, 118

cruciferous vegetables: how to get maximum immune function benefits of, 9; listed, 8, 159; recommended preparation, 8–10; recommended steaming times for, 10

crumbled spices, 36

cucumbers: ANDI score of, 28; "Dirty Dozen" pesticide level of, 39; herbs and spices to enhance flavor of, 180

cumin flavor, 36

Dates: Apple Supreme, 70; Berry Explosion Muffins, 76–77; comparing Medjool dates to Deglet Noor dates, 77; Crazy-For-Kale Salad with Dijon Pumpkin Seed Dressing, 134–135; Fudgy Black Bean Brownies, 283; Ginger Almond Dressing, 86, 309; Healthy Chocolate Cake, 286–287, 309; No-Bake Key Lime Pie, 293; Nutritarian Caesar Dressing, 82, 308; Quinoa Breakfast Pudding, 66; Red Velvet Sorbet, 305; Sesame Ginger Sauce, 108; Spiced Sweet Potato Cornbread, 266; Sweet Potato Peanut Chocolate Chip, 282; Ten Thousand Island Dressing, 87; Warm Spiced Butternut Squash Salad with Winesap Apples, 136–137

date sugar, 136–137

nutritarian tips (continued)
234; Native American mythology on the "three sisters," 167; never eat until you are full, 24; onions offer protection against diabetes, heart disease, and cancer, 118; recommended steaming times for green vegetables, 10; release anticancer compounds by chewing green vegetables, 139; on using tempeh, 237; unhealthful eating leads to food addictions, 62; vanilla bean to add flavor, 300; a word about food allergies, 21. *See also* Cooking to Live

nutrition: as most important building block of health, 1; studies on relationship between calories and, 1

nutritional ignorance: health consequences of, 2; misconceptions about olive oil, 26

nuts: allergy to, 21; benefits for coronary heart disease, 84; as source of good fat, 20–23; as super food, 29; tip on baking, 161; wide variety of, 22–23. *See also specific nuts; specific recipes*

Oak leaf lettuce–guide for using, 113

oatmeal: ANDI score of, 28; as whole grain food, 23

old-fashioned rolled oats: Banana Oat Bars, 284; Better Burgers, 250–251, 308; Cara's Apple Strudel, 285; Chia Cookies, 278–279; cooking chart for, 62; Goji Berry Walnut Squares with Chocolate Drizzle, 280–281; as whole grain food, 23. *See also* quick oats cooking chart

olive oil: ANDI score of, 28; misconceptions about, 26

onions: ANDI score of, 28; "Clean Fifteen" pesticide level of, 39; as G-BOMBS food, 22, 246; health benefits of, 9, 118; as super food, 29. *See also specific recipes*

orange ANDI score, 28

orange bell peppers, 94

oregano flavor, 36

organic produce, 38–39

Oswald, Martin, 42, 109, 136

Papayas, 16

paprika flavor, 36

parsley flavor, 36

peaches: ANDI score of, 28; "Dirty Dozen" pesticide level of, 39; Peach Apricot Sorbet, 303

peanut butter: ANDI score of, 28; Sweet Potato Peanut Chocolate Chip Cookies, 282

pears: how to pick a ripe, 16; Pomegranate Poached Pears with Chocolate and Raspberry Sauces, 298–299

peas. *See* green peas

pecans: Apple Berrynut Bites, 277; Artichoke Lentil Loaf, 204–205; Blueberry Nut Oatmeal, 63; Great Greens, 213; Pecan Cream, 305; Super Slaw, 119; Sweet Potato Black Bean Burgers, 252

persimmons: how to pick a ripe, 17; Persimmon Pud-

ding, 295; stir-fry classic menu inclusion of, 309. *See also specific recipes*

pesticides: "Clean Fifteen" produce lowest in, 39; "Dirty Dozen" produce highest in, 39

pesto tip, 109

phytosterols, 84

pies: Coconut Carrot Cream Pie, 288–289; No-Bake Key Lime Pie, 293; Pineapple Strawbana Pie, 292; Pumpkin Pie with Almond Crust, 290–291

pineapples: ANDI score of, 28; "Clean Fifteen" pesticide level of, 39; how to pick a ripe, 17; Pineapple Strawbana Pie, 292; Strawberry Pineapple Sorbet, 304, 309

pine nuts: Eggplant Cannelloni with Pine Nut Romesco Sauce, 194–195, 309; exceptional nutritional value of, 90; Mediterranean, 90, 195. *See also specific recipes*

pinto beans: Bean Enchiladas, 254, 308; Goji Chili Stew, 177; Sunny Bean Burgers, 249

pistachio nuts ANDI score, 28

pita bread: healthy "wrap" using, 248; Italian Stuffer, 258, 307; Pita/Tortilla Crisps, 103; Popeye Pitas with Mediterranean Tomato Spread, 259; Portobello Red Pepper Sandwich, 260; Roasted Vegetable Pizza, 257. *See also* whole-wheat products

plums: how to pick a ripe, 17; Mushroom and Chickpea Sofrito in Rainbow Chard with Spiced Plum Salad, 240–241

polycystic ovarian syndrome, 32

pomegranate juice ANDI score, 28

pomegranates: how to pick a ripe, 18; Pomegranate Poached Pears with Chocolate and Raspberry Sauces, 298–299; as super food, 29

Pomi brand, 9

portion-size measuring, 3

Positive Impact Magazine, 43

potatoes (white), 28, 39. *See also* sweet potatoes

poultry: ANDI score of chicken breast, 28; Black Bean Turkey Burgers, 274; Creole Chicken and Spinach, 273. *See also* meat

powered spices, 36

pressure cooker, 34

produce: "Clean Fifteen," 39; "Dirty Dozen," 39; organic, 39–40

Puck, Wolfgang, 42

puddings: Avocado Chocolate Pudding, 296; Mango Pudding, 294; Persimmon Pudding, 295

pumpkin seeds: Braised Kale and Squash with Pumpkin Seeds, 210; Crazy-For-Kale Salad with Dijon Pumpkin Seed Dressing, 134–135; as high-omega–3 fats source, 22, 23; Red Quinoa, Roasted Rainbow Carrots, Brussels Sprouts, Pearl Onions, and Dulse Salad with Pumpkin Seeds and Verjus, 242–243; Spiced Pumpkin Seed Cabbage Salad, 117; as super food, 29

Quick and easy dinner menu, 309
quick oats cooking chart, 62. *See also* old-fashioned rolled oats
quinoa: Quinoa Breakfast Pudding, 66; Quinoa Mango Salad, 124; Red Quinoa, Roasted Rainbow Carrots, Brussels Sprouts, Pearl Onions, and Dulse Salad with Pumpkin Seeds and Verjus, 242–243; Sicilian Stuffed Peppers, 202; as whole grain food, 23

Radicchio, 113
radishes: as anticancer food, 159; for dipping, 94; recommended preparation of, 8–9. *See also specific recipes*
raspberries: Detox Green Tea, 59; Pomegranate Poached Pears with Chocolate and Raspberry Sauces, 298–299; Red Velvet Sorbet, 305; as superfood, 11. *See also specific recipes*
raw vegetables: dipping, 94; weight-loss by eating, 10
recipes: breakfast, 61–77; desserts, 275–306; dips, chips, and sauces, 94–110; Fuhrman fast food, 247–266; main dishes, 180–246; nonvegan dishes, 267–274; salad dressings, 79–92; salads, 111–137; smoothies, blended salads, and juices, 47–60; soups and stews, 141–177
red bell peppers: for dipping, 94; Portobello Red Pepper Sandwich, 260; Roasted Vegetable Pizza, 257; as super food, 29; Watermelon Gazpacho, 174. *See also* bell peppers
red cabbage: as anticancer food, 159; recommended preparation of, 8–9
red cayenne pepper flavor, 36
red leaf lettuce: guide to using, 113; as super food, 29
red meat. *See* meat
red peppers, 132, 308
resistant starch, 19–20
rice: black, 23; brown, 23; Creamed Forest Kale over Wild Rice, 212; wild, 23. *See also* grain products
Rohrbacher, James C., 42, 102, 110, 126
romaine lettuce: ANDI score of, 28; for dipping, 94; guide to using, 113; as super food, 29
rosemary flavor, 100
rutabaga leaf, 8–9

Sage flavor, 36
salad dressings recipes: Almond Balsamic Vinaigrette, 81, 309; Banana Walnut Dressing, 83; Blueberry Pomegranate Dressing, 84; Crazy-For-Kale Salad with Dijon Pumpkin Seed Dressing, 134–135; Creamy Roasted Garlic Dressing, 88; creating your own, 80; Ginger Almond Dressing, 86, 309; Ginger-Poached Butternut Squash Salad with Warm Ginger Raisin Dressing, 138–139; Green Velvet Dressing, 85; Guacamole Dressing, 92, 308; Mixed Greens and Strawberry Salad, 114; Nutritarian Caesar Dressing, 82, 308; Orange Peanut Dressing, 89; Pesto

Salad Dressing, 90; recommended for weight-loss, diabetic, and metabolic syndrome, 93; Russian Fig Dressing, 91, 309; Spiced Pumpkin Seed Cabbage Salad, 117; Super Slaw, 119, 308; Taco Salad with Guacamole Dressing, 132, 308; Ten Thousand Island Dressing, 87; Warm Spiced Butternut Squash Salad with Winesap Apples, 136–137
salad recipes: Apple Bok Choy Salad, 116; Beluga Lentil Escabeche, 130; Chickpea "Tuno" Salad, 128–129; Crazy-For-Kale Salad with Dijon Pumpkin Seed Dressing, 134–135; Dijon Vinaigrette Asparagus, 120; guide to salad greens, 112–113; Jamaican Jerk Vegetable Salad, 127; Marinated Mushroom Salad, 121; Mixed Greens and Strawberry Salad, 114; Orange Sesame Micro Salad, 118, 307; Quinoa Mango Salad, 124; recommended for weight-loss, diabetic, and metabolic syndrome, 111; Salad of Roasted Beets and Asparagus with Black Cherry Vinaigrette, 122–123; Shredded Brussels Sprouts Salad, 115; Spiced Pumpkin Seed Cabbage Salad, 117; Super Slaw, 119, 308; Taco Salad with Guacamole Dressing, 132, 308; Three Bean Mango Salad, 125; Warm Braised Belgian Endive Salad with Raspberry Vinaigrette, 126; Warm Spiced Butternut Squash Salad with Winesap Apples, 136–137; Wild Rodeo Salad, 131; Wilted Arugula Milanese, 133. *See also* blended salads recipes
salmon: ANDI score of, 28; Salmon and Vegetables in a Packet, 272
salt-free seasoning blend recipe, 94
salt/sodium: avoid packaged food with high content of, 37; limiting intake of, 35–36; looking for labels on, 38
San Pellegrino World's 50 Best Restaurants survey, 42
sauce recipes: Arugula Pesto, 109; Blueberry Blast Sauce, 107; Brown Cremini Gravy, 105; Nutritarian Pickling Juice, 110; Sesame Ginger Sauce, 108; symbol indicating weight-loss, diabetic, and metabolic syndrome, 93; Tornado Tomato Sauce, 106
savory herbs, 36
seafood. *See* fish/seafood
seeds: as G-BOMBS food, 22, 246; as super food, 29; tip on baking, 161. *See also specific type of seed*
Serrano chili, 110
sesame seeds: ANDI score of, 28; as super food, 29
shrimp ANDI score, 28
smoothies recipes: Apple Oatberry Smoothie, 50; Berry Banana Smoothie, 49; Boston Green Smoothie, 54; Chocolate Cherry Smoothie, 52; infinite blending combinations for, 48; Pomegranate Refresher, 60; Purple Monster Smoothie, 56. *See also* blended salads
snow peas: pods for dipping, 94; recommended steaming times for, 10
sodium: avoid packaged food with high content of, 37; limiting intake of, 35–36; looking for labels on, 38

turnip greens: as anticancer food, 159; recommended preparation of, 8–9; as super food, 29
turnips, 94

USDA Choose My Plate, 30

Vanilla bean, 300, 301
vanilla ice cream ANDI score, 28
vegetable broth: Acorn Squash Stew with Brussels Sprouts, 145; Homemade Vegetable Broth, 144
vegetable juice, 90
vegetable juicer, 34
vegetables: allium, 9; cruciferous, 7–10, 159; dipping, 94; nutrients from, 7; recommended steaming times for green, 10; release anticancer compounds by chewing green, 139; starchy, 10; weight-loss by eating raw, 9. *See also specific vegetables*
VegiZest, 41. *See also specific recipes;* spices/herbs
vinegars. *See* Dr. Fuhrman's Favorite Vinegars
Vitamix blender, 34, 48

Walnuts: allergy to, 21; ANDI score of, 28; Banana Walnut Dressing, 83; Brussels Sprouts with Orange and Walnuts, 216; Goji Berry Walnut Squares with Chocolate Drizzle, 280–281; as high-omega–3 fats source, 20–23; as super food, 29
Waltermyer, Christine, 43–44
watercress: ANDI score of, 28; as anticancer food, 159; guide to using, 113; recommended preparation of, 8–9; as super food, 29

watermelon: causal backyard dinner with, 308; "Clean Fifteen" pesticide level of, 39; how to pick a ripe, 18; Watermelon Gazpacho, 174
water-sautéing (sweating or steam-frying), 33–34
weekly meal plan, 39–40
weight-loss diet: breakfast recipes recommended for a, 61; dips, chips, and sauces recipes recommended for a, 93; main dish recipes recommended for, 178–179; salad dressings recipes recommended for a, 79; salad recipes recommended for a, 111; smoothies, blended salads, and juices recipes recommended for a, 47; soups and stews recipes recommended for, 141
white bread ANDI score, 28
white pasta ANDI score, 28
white potatoes: ANDI score of, 28; "Dirty Dozen" pesticide level of, 39
whole-wheat products: ANDI score of bread, 28; choosing bread, 24; Healthy Chocolate Cake, 286–287, 309; healthy "wrap" materials, 248; spelt, 23. *See also* grain products; pita bread; tortillas
wild rice, 23
wrap sandwiches. *See* Fuhrman fast food recipes

Yellow bell peppers, 94

Zucchini: ANDI score of, 28; for dipping, 94; No-Pasta Zucchini Lasagna, 196–197; recommended steaming times for, 10. *See also specific recipes*

FOR MORE INFORMATION, VISIT:

. . . .

WWW.DRFUHRMAN.COM

Dr. Fuhrman's official website for information,
recipes, supportive services, and products.

or call:

(800) 474-WELL (9355)

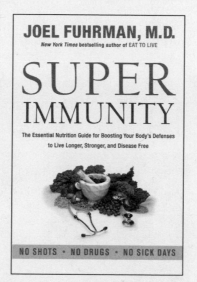
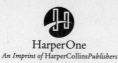

Also Available from HarperOne

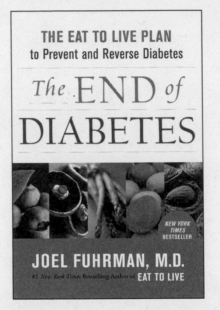

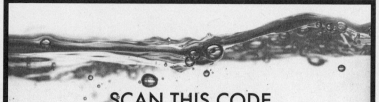

SCAN THIS CODE
WITH YOUR SMARTPHONE TO BE LINKED TO
THE BONUS MATERIALS FOR

EAT TO LIVE COOKBOOK

on the Elixir website,
where you can also find information about other
healthy living books and related materials.

YOU CAN ALSO TEXT

EATTOLIVE to READIT (732348)

to be sent a link to the Elixir website.